Defeat Your
Cravings™

THE BACK DOOR TO WEIGHT LOSS

Eight Simple Steps to Permanently Control Food
Cravings from an Author Who's Helped Almost
2,000 Clients Stop Overeating
– And Has More Than One Million Readers

DISCLAIMER

For educational purposes only. You are responsible for determining your own dietary, medical, and psychological needs. If you require assistance with this task, you must consult with a licensed physician, dietitian, psychologist, and/or other appropriately qualified and licensed professional. No medical, psychological, and/or nutritional advice is offered through this book. Even though the author is a licensed psychologist, he does not offer psychological services, psychological advice and/or psychological counsel in his role as author of this book. In particular, if you have ever been diagnosed with an eating disorder, you agree to not create your diet, food plan and/or any food rules without the input and approval of a psychiatrist, psychologist, and/or licensed dietician. You also acknowledge and agree that there are certain medical problems which may underlie unnaturally strong cravings which only a licensed physician can diagnose, treat, and cure. Defeat Your Cravings, LLC is only willing to license you the right to read and/or utilize this book in the event you agree with these terms. If you do not agree with these terms, please do not read the book, delete it from all electronic devices you own, and/or return it to your place of purchase for a full refund (where applicable).

THE BRAVE MAN
IS HE WHO
OVERCOMES
NOT ONLY HIS
ENEMIES
BUT HIS
PLEASURES.

Democritus

Table of
CONTENTS

My Outrageous Promise: Control Your Cravings Forever 7

Don't Take My Word for It – I Can Prove It.. 10

Introduction: Why One Weird Psychologist's Struggle
With Food Can Help You Defeat Your Cravings Forever 15

Consulting for Big Food and Advertising.. 20

Cravings Come from the Reptilian Brain (Which Doesn't Know Love)........24

40,000+ People Convinced Me to Stop "Loving Myself Thin" 26

Part 01
Quick Start to Get Results Fast 29

How to Use This Book... 30

Step 01
Know Your Enemy.. 31

Step 02
Eliminate Your Enemy's Excuses.. 59

Part 02
Enhancing and Speeding Up the Process 71

Step 03
Turn Off the False Alarms 72

Step 04
Cultivate Powerful Motivation 90

Step 05
Extinguish Your Cravings 107

Step 06
Automate Motivation at the Moment of Impulse 118

Step 07
Have a Recovery Plan 137

Step 08
Build Community Support 147

From the Bottom of My Heart to the Bottom of Yours 155

Appendix 157

Appendix A: How To Refute the Most Common Squeals 158

Appendix B: What If It Doesn't Work? 171

Appendix C: Drugs and Alcohol 176

Appendix D: References 178

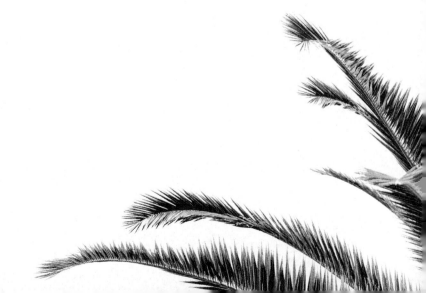

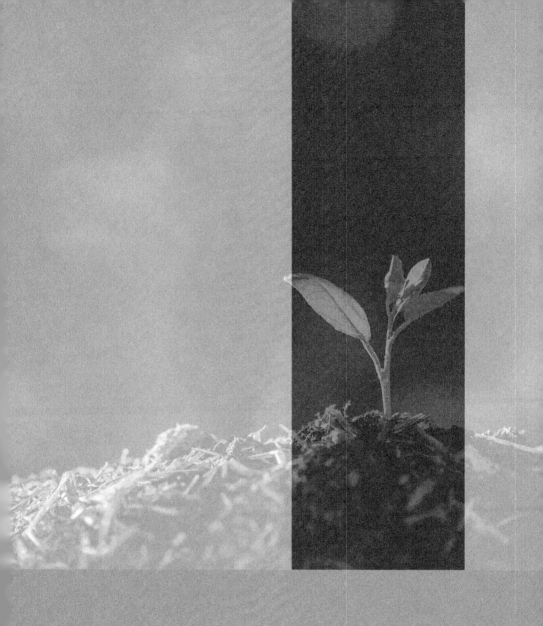

MY OUTRAGEOUS PROMISE

Control Your Cravings Forever

If you struggle with food in any way, from occasionally eating beyond your own best thinking to regularly consuming mass quantities, I'd like to make you an outrageous promise. Suspend judgment long enough to absorb a few unusual techniques and insights, and you can control your cravings forever. I'm not talking about white-knuckle, hold-on-for-your-life control, but rather the kind you can maintain indefinitely without constant attention and thought.

Do what I suggest step-by-step, and you can:

- ☑ Dramatically reduce those "impossible to resist" cravings which seem to come out of nowhere and derail your best-laid plans.
- ☑ Minimize damage from missteps and recover twice as fast.
- ☑ Reclaim five to ten hours per week formerly wasted on recovering from overeating.
- ☑ Reduce the frequency with which you give in to cravings by 85%+.
- ☑ Develop 100% confidence in your ability to maintain control forever, regardless of how many times you've tried before, and how far down you've slid into a personal food nightmare!
- ☑ Have significantly more energy and zest for life.
- ☑ Feel more mindful and present throughout your day.
- ☑ Think about food less than half as much as you do now.
- ☑ See how to steadily approach your ideal weight without being tortured by the diet mentality.
- ☑ Start saving thousands of dollars annually on junk food, restaurant deliveries, and other overeating behaviors.
- ☑ Feel like the master of your own fate with your food and your life.
- ☑ Learn to apply these tools to other disciplines – exercise, clutter, finance management, parenting, productivity, and work performance.

Plus, because this solution is entirely information-based, you won't need invasive surgery, side-effects-prone medication, or hundreds of hours on a therapist's couch.

I know it's probably hard to believe where you stand right now, but you also won't need to rely on willpower because you'll learn to make these eating patterns a natural part of who you are. And provided you avoid extreme diets and reliably eat enough nutritious food; you can defeat your cravings on the food plan of *your* choice. Low carb, high carb, plant-based, carnivore, point counting, calorie counting – it's up to you.

Lastly, *Defeat Your Cravings* is a formula for taking control of those "irresistible" urges that derail you from goals and dreams in all life areas. You can use this same formula for a multitude of positive pursuits like exercise, parenting, finances, work, friendship, romance, productivity, and more!

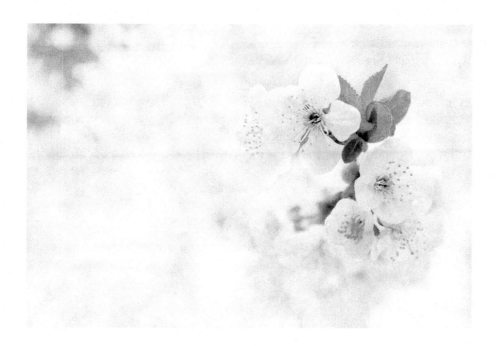

DON'T TAKE MY WORD FOR IT – I CAN PROVE IT

You don't need to take my word for any of this because I've got proof. So, please excuse my immodesty while I walk you through it.

In the past decade, I've worked with almost 2,000 overeaters in group and individual programs. In the last three of those years, we got serious about measuring results. Most clients engaged with their coaches at least every other day *("engaged client")* and reduced their problem eating by an average of 89.4% during the first month! This is the *typical* result for engaged clients during the past three years, *not* a statistical outlier or anecdotal testimonial.

Those who did not engage were in the minority, and, as you might expect, achieved little if any results. The overwhelming reason for not engaging in the program was *shame*, which we call "the overeater's curse," and we spent a great deal of time trying to overcome it. Eventually we understood that this mindset naturally lifts when you understand that cravings are almost always a normal, healthy function of the human brain.

In fact, those who struggle more with cravings may have been *better* suited for survival during 99.9% of the time human beings have been on the planet—before industry perverted our food supply. See, people who struggle with strong food cravings *(and overeating)* aren't sick, diseased, or broken. Mostly, these individuals are just people with healthy appetites that have been hijacked by Big Food for a profit. Of course, check with a physician to rule out physical causes, but I find the vast majority of "out-of-control" cravings are just the brain doing what it *thinks* you need do to survive in the modern food environment.

The fact that these methods worked so well is probably why my first book has almost 20,000 reviews on Amazon *(that's more than "The Da Vinci Code" by Dan Brown)* and nearly 1 million readers. In fact, it may be the most read book in the world on overeating.

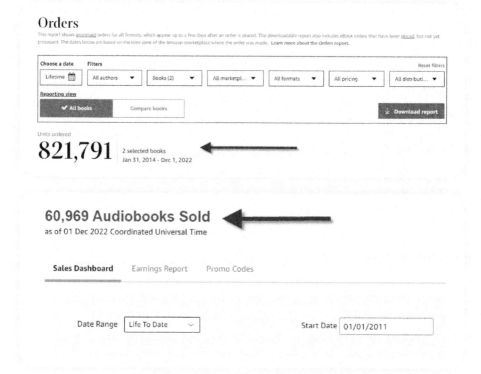

But there's something important you need to understand about the first book: It was written and published in 2015, and only modestly updated since. In contrast, this book, Defeat Your Cravings, is a comprehensive update of everything I know about cravings and overeating, intended to entirely replace the first.

Defeat Your Cravings contains wisdom derived from years of painstaking work in the trenches, evidence-based techniques, and scientific research.

Plus, while the first book was written for people who felt desperately addicted to food, *Defeat Your Cravings* is for *everyone*. You don't have to be a food addict to benefit. If you sometimes overeat due to strong cravings, you should find tremendous relief here. Of course, if you *are* addicted to food, this book can save you too.

For all these reasons, you'll find my best thinking in *Defeat Your Cravings (this book)*.

Now, if the results from my previous coaching programs and the popularity of the first book aren't enough to convince you, I've also written dozens of articles for *Psychology Today – one of the most popular websites in the world –* where I obtained an additional million readers:

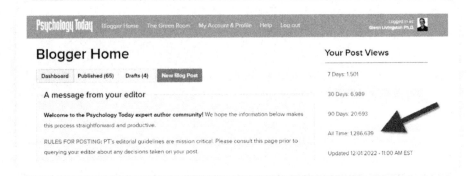

Plus, research, work, and theories from earlier in my career have been seen in dozens of periodicals and newspapers, on TV and radio, and in literally hundreds of podcasts worldwide:

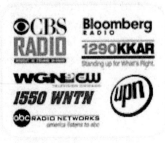
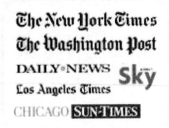

Okay, sorry for bragging, but it was necessary to cut through the noise of so many charlatans in the diet industry making unsupportable claims, and to open your mind to the possibility this approach will help.

There's one more reason this book is worth your while: The insights and techniques contained in these pages are entirely consistent with how the brain works. Many of the insights I'll share are so obviously common sense that you'll want to slap yourself in the head with a spatula wondering why you didn't already think of them before. *(But please don't do that because it's not your fault, and spatulas can leave permanent marks.)*

The reason people don't know how to defeat their cravings, stop overeating, and dramatically reduce their constant thinking about food is that all the mythology in our culture hides the truth. There are entire industries whose very existence depends on you not knowing it!

Big Food spends hundreds of millions of dollars to engineer hyper-palatable concentrations of starch, sugar, fat, salt, and excitotoxins, all targeting the bliss point in your reptilian brain without giving you enough nutrition to feel satisfied. This industry is pressing our hardwired, biological buttons with precision and force. Then Big Advertising spends a fortune to convince you that you need to consume these concoctions.

The result? Every time you bury your head in a bag, box, or container, some corporate fat cat in a white suit with a mustache is laughing all the way to the bank. Plus, at most social gatherings people tacitly support each other to slowly kill themselves with food while casually laughing it off together. "Everything in moderation!" "Just hand over the chocolate and nobody gets hurt!" Etc.

It's actually not funny though because, according to the Center for Disease Control and Prevention, 73.6% of adults are overweight in the United States. That's almost three out of four people! (CDC 2023) And:

- ☑ Worldwide obesity since 1975 has TRIPLED according to the World Health Organization (2021). More than 1.9 billion adults are overweight and 650,000,000 are obese.

- ☑ More than three times as many people live with diabetes (World Health Organization 2023). 108 million in 1980, and 422 million in 2014!

Diabetic adults live with double the risk of heart attack and stroke. They also have a seriously increased risk of blindness and kidney failure. Yet: "Keeping weight in check, being active, and eating a healthy diet can help prevent most cases of type 2 diabetes," according to Harvard University's School of Public Health (Harvard 2023).

- ☑ Cardiovascular disease is responsible for 32% of global deaths. (World Health Organization 2021)

- ☑ But, "Most cardiovascular disease can be prevented by addressing behavioral risk factors – primarily unhealthy diet, obesity, and lack of exercise."

- ☑ 30% to 40% of cancers might be prevented by diet and lifestyle alone (Donaldson 2004).

To make matters worse, whether through the airwaves or the internet, every year thousands of food advertisements bombard us, almost none of which are about eating more whole foods. This year, the packaged foods market is valued at $2.9 trillion dollars (Verified Market Research 2023), whereas the global market for fresh produce is less than five percent of this (Market Data Forecast 2023). As you might expect, there's not much profit in advertising produce, as the big bucks are in packaged goods.

Now, most people think advertising doesn't affect them, but did you know it affects you more when you think that because it lowers your sales resistance? The industry has us exactly where they want us!

All of the above creates a perfect storm for out-of-control cravings and weight gain. But the good news is, you can take control and stop overeating without becoming diet-obsessed. Just eliminate the mythology and define what healthy eating means to you personally. Take a long, hard look at the truth, make some up-front decisions, and learn some straightforward, practical techniques. That's what this book is about. You *can* defeat your cravings, lose weight, and stop suffering. And the best part is, you can get most of the work done in 30 days!

I don't say this lightly because I know how much can be at stake if you're caught in the grips of strong, destructive food cravings. On my mother's grave, I promise. *(Don't worry, Mom, I've got you covered!)*

But first, let me tell you a little more about myself.

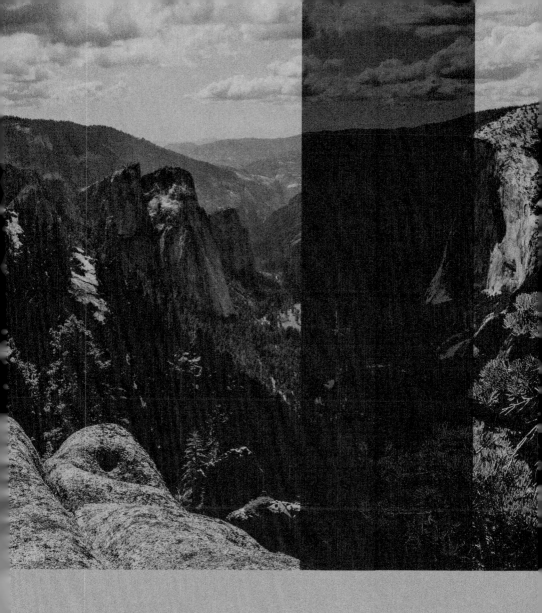

INTRODUCTION

Why One Weird Psychologist's
Struggle With Food Can Help You
Defeat Your Cravings Forever

Download the FREE Reader Bonuses:
This book comes with a full set of materials intended to enrich and enhance its use. Download them FREE at
www.DefeatYourCravings.com

- ☑ **A One-Page Cheat-Sheet for the Entire *Defeat Your Cravings Process*...**

- ☑ **Free Food Plan Starter Templates with Step-by-Step Customization:** Pre-filled starter templates to use *Defeat Your Cravings* on *any* diet —keto, whole foods plant based, point counting, calorie counting, etc. Step-by-step instructions to customize it for your own needs!

- ☑ **Practical Takeaways from the Science of Cravings Extinction Cheat Sheet:** Discover the best ways to dramatically downgrade your cravings, fast! *(Cheat Sheet.)*

- ☑ **The "Abstinence vs. Moderation" Cheat Sheet:** "Must I give it up or can I still eat some?" Most can moderate but some need to abstain. It differs by person and by treat. See where you fall!

- ☑ Overcoming F.O.M.O. *(the "Fear of Missing Out")* Cheat Sheet: Don't let your lower-food-self talk you into overeating just because everyone else is!

- ☑ **How to Turn Off the False Alarms That Drive Overeating:** Ever suffer from a case of the *"Screw It, Just Do Its!?"* Try this...

- ☑ **Craving Defeater Set:** Quickly defeat ANY craving! Print it out and carry it around with you, and keep the MP3 audio on your smart phone ...

- ☑ **The Overeating Episode Recovery Set:** How to reactivate your higher-food-self after overeating. Stop the episode from getting worse! *(Audios and Cheat Sheets)* ...

- ☑ **Unusual Ways to Neutralize Other People's Pigs:** Troubled by what other people say, do, or tempt you with in an eating environment? Neutralize their power! *(Audio and Transcript)* ...

- ☑ **The "No Regrets" Worksheet:** How to see the road not taken: "To indulge or not to indulge. That is the question!" The two different paths and where they may lead.

- ☑ **Overeating Damage Calculator:** Get a good hard look at reality to boost your motivation...

- ☑ **Common Food Industry Lies (and How to Defeat Them):** Here are some tricky ways they get you, and simple strategies for winning the game! *(Audio Interview + Transcript)* ...

- ☑ **Smart Phone App and Free Reader's Community:** Connect with others for support, get audios, videos, and access to webinars not available elsewhere!

Download Them All for FREE at:
www.DefeatYourCravings.com

Clients and readers of my previous book please note: If you already know and trust me, you can safely skip this introduction and begin with Part One. Even if you are familiar with my previous work, however, you should still read Part One, because there are some significant updates included which lay a stronger foundation for the rest of the process. That said, you will find that Part Two contains most of the newer findings and contributes several additional pieces and parts to the puzzle, which make the method much more effective. (*The motivational section is the only part of Part Two that you'll largely recognize from my previous work, but it, too, has been updated.*)

I'm not just the author, but a success story myself. In the next few pages, I'll summarize my quest to defeat my own cravings and lay the foundation for how you can do it about 100 times faster than I did. "I wish I knew then what I know now," etc.

So, have you ever been to the Woodbury Country Deli in Syosset, New York? If you visited in the 90s, you might've found them out of muffins, pizza, soda, and chocolate if I got there before you!

I'm a formerly obese psychologist previously obsessed with food at a truly humiliating level. I lost a war with a chocolate bar somewhere around 1982, then spent decades buried under a mountain of bags, boxes, and containers. I couldn't stop thinking about food even when sitting with suicidal patients. Thankfully, I never lost anyone.

Chocolate was my worst enemy, but I also ate mounds of pasta, pizza, muffins, donuts, and pretty much anything else which wasn't nailed down! Therefore, please know this book is not only about chocolate cravings, despite the fact I talk about them a lot. They're just a good illustration. The same process works for *any* craving, as we've subsequently proven with so many clients.

My struggle began as an adolescent. I'm six-foot-four and the genetic lottery blessed me with a modestly muscular frame – at seventeen I could eat whatever I wanted if I worked out for two hours per day. A half dozen chocolate bars, a whole pizza (*or two*), boxes of muffins, boxes of donuts, soda, two plates of pasta, a box of cookies, etc. At the time, I thought this was super cool. I guess that's why they say, "Youth is wasted on the young."

I got away with eating like this until about the age of 22. At that point, I was married and had begun commuting two hours each way to see patients and take classes for my Ph.D. At night, I had to help my wife with her business; so, I could no longer find two minutes per day to exercise, much less two hours. My metabolism slowed, too, but the more critical factor was that food seemed to have taken on a life of its own. I couldn't adjust my intake. It had a real hold on me.

At first, I didn't gain much weight, but the constant cravings interfered with my ability to be fully present with patients. I come from a family of seventeen therapists, so being a great psychologist has always been most important to me. My mom, dad, sister, stepfather, stepmother, grandmother, cousins, uncle, aunt, and great uncles and aunts are *all* therapists. When something broke in the house, we all knew how to ask it how it felt but nobody knew how to fix it. At nine years old, I'd take my little friends down to my father's office in the basement, tell them to lie down on the couch, and tell me about their mothers. I wish I were kidding.

What I learned quickly from being a doctor in the mental health space is that it *wasn't* all about solving the jigsaw puzzle of your patient's life from your years of accumulated knowledge and training. It also involved getting your client to love and trust you enough to stretch their comfort zone, think new thoughts, and try new behaviors. This required unwavering presence – *I had to lend them my soul* – and food was distracting me. I had to find a solution.

Coming from the family I came from you might not be surprised that I chose the depth-psychology route to deal with my food problems. "There must be a hole in my heart," I reasoned, "and if I could fill that, I wouldn't have to keep filling the hole in my stomach." So, I embarked on a 20-year quest to love myself thin.

I saw the best psychologists and psychiatrists in the New York City area. I recited chapter and verse about my childhood, my earliest romantic experiences, my traumas, mishaps, and adventures. I cried. I screamed. I confessed all the things a good little neurotic Jewish boy needed to confess to cleanse his soul. I learned a lot about myself. It was, in fact, a very enriching journey and I don't regret one moment of it. Unfortunately, it was also accompanied by *even more* chocolate, pasta, pizza, muffins, and donuts!

You see, no matter which approach I tried, I'd get a little thinner, then a lot fatter. Over the years – *despite the personal psychological and spiritual growth* – my cravings, overeating, and food obsession only worsened. At my lowest point, I was likely near 300 pounds, though I don't know that number for sure since I stopped weighing myself when I reached 257 pounds. My triglycerides peaked at 1,000+ and my doctors warned me I was going to die at a young age. I had psoriasis, rosacea, and eczema. It's not an exaggeration to say my cravings were destroying all of me – body, mind, and soul.

Thankfully, toward the end of 2007, several profound insights shook my confidence in the "love yourself thin approach," which I finally came to realize wasn't working for me. Instead, I pivoted to a "be the alpha-wolf of your own mind" paradigm, an approach I decided to try after learning first-hand about the food and advertising industries and their sophisticated tactics to deceive the consumer.

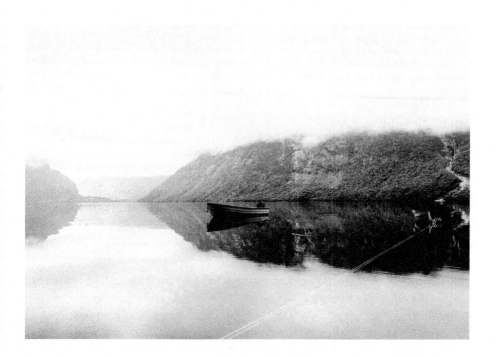

CONSULTING FOR BIG FOOD AND ADVERTISING

Ironically, I'm a child and family psychologist who never had children because I married a woman who traveled for business. This, and working from home, gave me oodles of time for a second career, so in addition to my clinical practice, I became CEO of a multi-million-dollar advertising research firm. Our clients were mostly in the Big Food and Big Pharma industries. I worked with many executives firsthand.

I know now I was on the wrong side of the war. I feel guilty about the work I did back then, and I'm now working very hard to make up for it. At the time, I'd fooled myself into believing I'd eventually rise to a position of influence and get these companies to change. I thought their respect for me would outweigh the mountain of profit they made from selling sugar to kids. Well, at one time I also thought Barbara Eden from *I Dream of Jeannie* was going to come to my house, blink her eyes, and vaporize the kids at school I didn't like. You might say, as a young man, I was prone to fantasy.

I did learn important things working with the food industry though. For example, I saw the millions of dollars they spent to stimulate cravings and discovered it had almost nothing to do with our personal psychology. For example, I thought I had to heal my depression, loneliness, and other emotional conflicts before I could fix my food problem, but the industry dispelled this notion for me. How could a therapist's advice stand a chance against a food supply that was being engineered to turn on my cravings and turn off my ability to know when I was full?

Toward the end of my consulting days, I did a very potent thought experiment: I asked myself if I believed there were such things as overeating and food addiction 100,000 years ago. My answer was that I didn't think Thag sat around the campfire holding his stomach saying, *"Oy Marta! Eat way too much mammoth!"* This made it clear that modern-day cravings were a byproduct of what industry had done to our food supply, not a mysterious psychological disease, disorder, or condition. The industry created cravings using knowledge of human physiology and the brain, no matter what "old tapes" from childhood I might've been replaying.

Maybe this "mom didn't love you enough" theory wasn't all it was cracked up to be!

I also realized the culprit wasn't only Big Food. Big Advertising excelled at making everyone think they needed these hyper-palatable, food-like substances. They tapped into our survival drive and stimulated the brain on a primitive level with *their* methods too.

For example, in nature, a diverse set of colors signals the availability of a diverse set of nutrients. A salad with dark green romaine lettuce, rich blue blueberries, deep red tomatoes, bright orange carrots, and purple cabbage provides a lot more nutrition when compared to a simple bowl of iceberg lettuce. For this reason, humans have evolved a "variety impulse" to keep eating in response to varied color. It's an almost automatic biological reflex, and believe me, Big Food knows this, and often uses multicolored, vibrant wrappers regardless of the nutrition level in their products. *(Marketers also know color can influence more than 62% of people's attitude toward a given product or brand (Sing 2006). Also see Paakki et al. (2019) regarding the use of color saturation, depth, and contrast to create food attraction. Women may be more sensitive to food color, especially when hungry (Chao et al. 2017).)*

Chip manufacturers leverage the variety impulse in a different way. They may use a multitude of assembly lines for each bag, each with a slightly different flavored chip because, in nature, a patch of food with varied taste also signals an increased presence of diverse micronutrients.

Then there's the phenomenon of "plausible deniability." The food industry has discovered people only need to believe they're eating healthily to justify purchase. For example, most people associate avocados with health, so you might see a great big "Made with Avocado Oil" star on a package of chips, ignoring the fact *any* oil heated at high temperatures can be carcinogenic, as are the acrylamides formed in the baking process. Also, there's almost no nutrition in chips. In your heart of hearts, you knew that, right? But the star on the label lets you think "at least they're healthy" as you scarf down a bag or two *(or three, or four)*. Plausible deniability is all the justification the rational brain needs to allow indulgence.

Please don't get the wrong idea about what I'm preaching. I believe we all have the right to eat potato chips if we want to. In fact, in two out of three cases, I find it's unnecessary for people to abstain from their favorite junk food once they know how to regulate it. But you can get yourself in a lot of trouble *pretending* things are healthy when they're not. There's also a big difference between believing something is less bad for you versus convincing yourself it's good for you. If you want to indulge, indulge. Just don't pretend.

Later, I'll go into detail about effective techniques for indulging with clear boundaries to minimize harm. The important point is, Big Advertising and Big Food engage in perfectly legal, predatory practices which stimulate cravings and food obsession, and these powerful economic forces exert their influence independent of our personal psychology.

Intriguingly, predation in industry mimics predation in nature. In his book *Influence, The Psychology of Persuasion,* Robert Cialdini presents a complex relationship between three species of fish. One, let's call it "Charlie," tends to get a lot of seaweed stuck in its teeth. Hey, it happens, don't judge! But thankfully nature has provided Charlie with a "Joe" fish who likes to clean his teeth. When he's in a teeth-cleaning mood, Joe does a special little dance to put Charlie into a trance so he can do his job. It's a grand fish-flossing contract in a world where dental floss doesn't exist. Win-win.

Enter a third species I'll call "Hector." Hector has learned to *mimic* Joe's dance. He can put Charlie into a trance too, except Hector has evil intent. Hector trances Charlie, not to get the seaweed from between his teeth, but so he can feast on the flesh in Charlie's mouth. Not such a great day at the hygienist for Charlie.

We're the Charlie fish. Big Food and Big Advertising are Hectors. It's enough to make you think twice about those chips, isn't it?

The point is the industry pushes brain buttons regardless of any psychological trauma, personality, or neurotic guilt you may be carrying from childhood. Big Food and Big Advertising excel at making you believe their products support your survival needs, but it's mostly just a trick. No doctor is going to diagnose you with a potato chip deficiency.

Strike two for the "love yourself thin" approach.

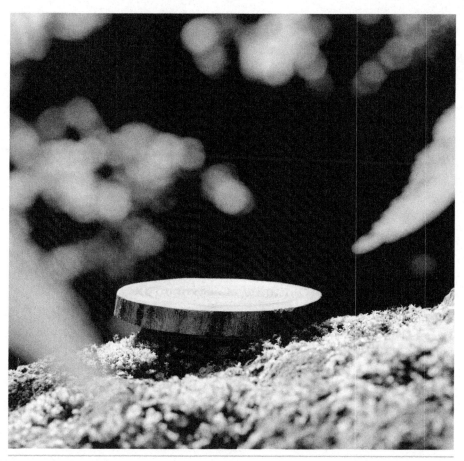

CRAVINGS COME FROM THE REPTILIAN BRAIN
(WHICH DOESN'T KNOW LOVE)

In 1989, I learned something in neuropsychology class which I unfortunately proceeded to ignore for decades: The "reptilian brain" (*brain stem*) is where our survival drives live. Fight or flight, feast or famine, reproduce or turn away. When the reptilian brain encounters something new in the environment, it asks itself: *"Do I eat it, mate with it, or kill it?"*

Love is notably absent from this example because it requires higher brain functions to delay action while considering the impact on others. *"Hey! Before you eat, mate, or kill that thing, how will it affect your family, tribe, or herd?"*

Longer-term goals like weight loss and fitness require even higher brain functions. *"Before you do anything, how will it impact your goals and dreams?"*

Cravings mostly seem to arise from the primitive feast-or-famine function, which can override higher brain functions when it *perceives* an emergency or detects the opportunity to gather scarce resources. That's why your best judgment goes out the window when you're in front of that chocolate bar, bagel, or donut. In hindsight, it was fruitless to spend decades trying to love myself thin because the reptilian brain doesn't know love. Sigh.

Today there is some controversy about exactly where these brain functions are located. What's not controversial, though, is the fact they *exist*, and that the lower-level functions can push aside our rational minds in a perceived emergency. Therefore, please don't get caught up in the anatomical structure. The higher-self versus lower-self may be more widely distributed in the brain than we believed in 1989. What matters is, you can take steps to return control to the higher, more rational self when you detect the lower self has taken over.

For similar reasons, it also doesn't matter whether these functions evolved or not, or if God put them there. The techniques in this book work independently of your religion, faith, or lack thereof.

All you really need to know is there's a higher brain function (*"higher self"*) which uses logic and reason to pursue those goals to which we've rationally committed, and a lower function (*"lower self"*) which pushes aside our best thinking and says, *"Screw it, just eat,"* when it thinks it's found valuable food resources or perceives urgent action is required.

Alas, while I knew this in 1989, I didn't put two and two together. Instead, I continued my psychological quest for decades, burying myself under a mountain of bags, boxes, and containers.

Until...

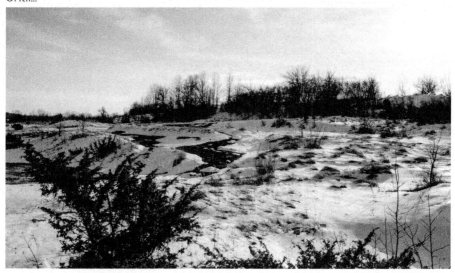

40,000+ PEOPLE CONVINCED ME TO STOP "LOVING MYSELF THIN"

In the late 90s, when internet clicks were cheap, I decided to fund a big online survey to study the relationship between cravings and stress. For approximately five years, I intercepted people searching for help with stress and asked them what they were most stressed about, and what kinds of foods they struggled with when they felt this way. Three intriguing findings emerged:

- ☑ People who craved chocolate (*like me*) tended to be stressed by loneliness, a broken heart, or depression.
- ☑ Those who craved soft, chewy, starchy things like pasta, pizza, and bagels tended to be stressed at home.
- ☑ People who craved salty, crunchy foods such as chips and pretzels tended to be stressed at work.

I thought these were profound insights, but at the time I was very busy with other things and didn't explore them much further. I put the study on the back burner for years.

Eventually, a little after turning forty *(I'm almost 60 now)*, I was complaining about my food struggles to my mother. For some reason we started talking about this study and I asked her how it might apply to my upbringing.

"Mom, why do I turn to chocolate when I feel lonely, broken hearted, or depressed? Do you remember when that all started?"

Her voice took on a horrible tone of shame. I'll never forget it.

"I'm so sorry, Glenn. So very, very sorry," she said.

"Mom, it's okay. It was decades ago. I love you. I forgive you. I just want to understand!"

"Well, when you were one year old in 1965, I was trying to get pregnant with your sister and your dad was a Captain in the Army. They wanted to send him to Vietnam, and I was terrified. Around the same time, your grandfather had just reappeared after disappearing for two years, and we had no idea where he had been. I'd always idolized him, and didn't know he was doing illegal things, but he was, and I was devastated. I became *extremely* depressed and anxious, and mostly just sat around staring at the wall. So, I didn't have the wherewithal to take care of you. I didn't play with you, hug you, and love you the way I should have. Instead, I got a big bottle of Bosco chocolate syrup and put it in a little refrigerator on the floor. When you needed something, I'd say, 'Go get your Bosco, Glenn,' and you'd go crawl over to the fridge, open the cap, suck on the bottle, and enter a chocolate-sugar coma for a few hours. I created a 'Bosco babysitter' and I'm so ashamed."

While Mom was horrified, I was excited because now it suddenly all made sense. After all these years I finally knew what caused my problem. If this were a movie, Mom and I would've had a big hug and a big cry, and that would've been the end of my chocolate struggles forever!

Well, we did have a metaphorical hug *(on Skype)*, and I felt a great sense of psychological relief. I thought I'd finally loved myself out of the problem. Unfortunately, the exact opposite happened. My cravings got worse, and I was devastated. Little did I know that as compelling as the psychological insight seemed, this experience would be what finally convinced me I couldn't "love myself thin." It eventually led to the first component of the method to defeat your cravings for good. If you'd told me back then that millions of people would be using it now, I would have dismissed it completely. But as I've learned, truth can be stranger than fiction.

Let's get started with the work in earnest!

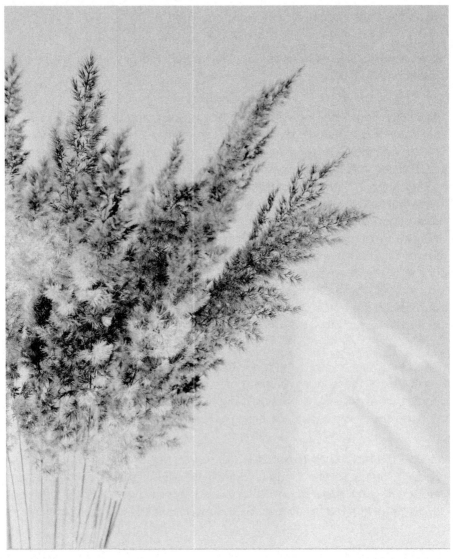

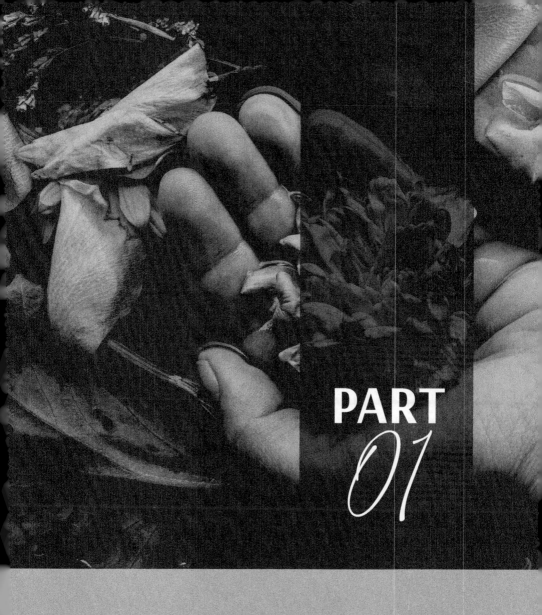

PART
01

QUICK START TO
GET RESULTS FAST

HOW TO USE THIS BOOK

Each of the eight steps in the *Defeat Your Cravings* methods will take some learning and practice to implement correctly. A full implementation of every step is *not* required to defeat every undesirable craving or eating habit. Some respond to just the first one or two steps whereas others require all eight. Especially after the first two steps, it's important not to get stuck trying to perfect any given one. You'll come back to each step over time and get better and better at it. Getting started is what's most important!

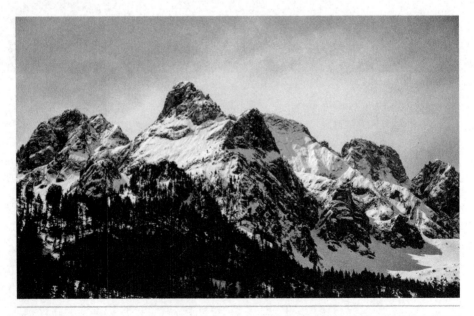

KNOW YOUR ENEMY

The conversation with Mom was helpful. Understanding the origin of my cravings led to a lot more compassion for both of us. We learned more about each other. It drew us closer.

But something inside me latched on to this story as an excuse to indulge *more*. A distinct, repetitive thought emerged: *"Hey, Glenn, you were right! Your mom didn't love you enough. She left a great big chocolate-sized hole in your heart and, until you fix the marriage or find true love, you've got to keep filling it with chocolate. Otherwise, you'll be tortured with cravings forever; so, there's no point resisting. Go get some now, you fool. Omnonmnomnom! Yippee!"*

No, I'm not schizophrenic. Everyone lives with an internal voice of justification. Mine just got *a lot* stronger once it got a hold of this story.

Now, I should reveal something at this juncture which is embarrassing for a psychologist with my credentials and experience, because my first insight into defeating my cravings was extremely rude and crude. Remember, I wasn't planning on teaching it. It was just a desperate attempt to find personal relief. I had no idea this would become so widespread and popular. So, I really hope you'll give the rest of this book a chance, regardless of your initial reaction. I promise, I've made this method *much* less abrasive over the years, and you do *not* have to do it as I did.

So, here it is: I decided to call my reptilian brain my inner "Pig." Then I made rules like, *"I'll never eat chocolate on a weekday again,"* to separate my own thoughts about eating from those of the Pig. For example, anything suggesting I should hold steady and not give in to weekday chocolate temptation was my higher self; everything else was my Pig. I called the Pig's thoughts "Squeals," and food on the wrong side of the line was "Slop."

For example, I might be at Starbucks on Wednesday when a chocolate bar beckoned at the checkout counter, and I'd observe myself thinking, *"You worked out hard today! You won't gain any weight if you eat some chocolate. Just a few bites won't hurt you even though it's Wednesday. Besides, it'll be just as easy to start again tomorrow."*

With the new technique in place, I'd think...

Whoa! Wait a minute! Chocolate on a weekday is Pig Slop! I don't eat Pig Slop and I don't let farm animals tell me what to do!

Ridiculous? Yes.

Classy? No.

Effective? Yes!

Self-Abuse? Well, I could've used a different word, and you should feel free to do so if the term "Pig" bothers you. But this was the first method that really worked to wake me up at the moment of impulse and give me those few extra microseconds to make a better decision. It inserted a long enough pause to remember my commitment.

It wasn't a miracle cure, but it was progress! I no longer felt there was some mysterious, unidentifiable force at work "forcing" me to eat. I stopped wasting my life trying to "love myself thin." I more frequently recognized when my lower self was active, and because of this awareness I had more opportunity to make better choices. Period, end of story.

The separation and ability to pause before giving in to my cravings made it possible to examine my excuses for indulgence *(the Squeals)* more thoroughly. For example, when the Pig said, *"It'll be just as easy to start again tomorrow,"* I'd say, *"No it won't, Pig!"* The way the brain works, if you have a craving, then think "start again tomorrow," and then indulge, you'll reinforce both the craving *and* the thought. My craving will be worse tomorrow, and I'll be more likely to have the same thought again. I always use the present moment to be healthy. When I'm in a hole I need to stop digging!

In hindsight, without this heightened awareness, nothing else mattered because my lower self could too easily push aside my best thinking when I had a craving. Before this clear separation, I'd always felt like I'd been hit by a runaway truck. There wasn't enough time and space to figure out what was going on! It's like the food was in my mouth the moment the craving hit. But armed with this new awareness, it became possible to pause and reflect on my lower-self's arguments without acting on them. That's why this approach made such a dramatic difference.

Over the years, having the ability to separate myself from the cravings and take the time to pause gave me the space to develop additional techniques. Without this pause, virtually nothing else worked because there wasn't enough time and space to operate.

Depending upon how serious the craving and associated food behavior is, separation *can* be enough in and of itself to fix the problem. That said, the additional *Defeat Your Cravings* techniques in the chapters ahead are vital additions. They dramatically speed up the process of leaving cravings in the past and are often required to defeat difficult ones. The separation technique is always necessary, but often not sufficient. The additional skills we layer on top of separation include:

- ☑ Logically disempowering enemy excuses for indulgence *(Squeals)*.
- ☑ Improving motivation *and* programming it to reflexively "pop up" when cravings hit.
- ☑ Implementing four simple ways to turn off the "false alarms" in your brain which create the "screw it, just do it" response – where your rational thinking gets pushed aside and it seems like all that matters is giving in.
- ☑ Actively improving nutrition and redirecting the cravings toward healthier alternatives.
- ☑ Severing the link between emotional upset and overeating.
- ☑ Eliminating excess guilt and shame. *(These emotions only perpetuate cravings and lead to more destructive food behavior.)*
- ☑ Becoming more mindful when you eat.
- ☑ Reducing food obsession.

Taken together, these skills form the *Defeat Your Cravings* method. Properly applied, there's virtually no craving or food behavior you can't beat. Adopting this approach will radically alter your relationship with food after just a brief period of study and practice. In fact, you might not recognize yourself in 30 days! The rest of this book lays out the process in detail, including how to customize it for your personal dietary plan.

Let's start by crafting *one simple rule*. Choose something not too onerous but that will still make a big difference. Your first goal is to restore your sense of power, hope, and enthusiasm so you can experience at least a modest win in an arena which has likely beaten you down for a long time. Then, you'll leverage that momentum to power through the rest of the way.

Before creating your rule, however, I'll show you how to overcome some common objections to food rules themselves, as well as objections to clearly separating the thoughts of your higher versus lower self so you can begin to put your food cravings into context.

OVERCOMING COMMON OBJECTIONS

The thought-separating technique and the use of food rules grate against many commonly held cultural beliefs. Objections are to be expected. Within the answers to these objections are several core principles that are necessary for success. In fact, most people say the answers to these objections are powerful and unexpected, even *(and perhaps especially)* when they didn't have a particular objection in the first place.

Some common objections include:

- ☑ Using the word "Pig" may encourage self-abuse.
- ☑ Incorporating food rules may *cause* overeating.
- ☑ Adopting this approach will make me a perfectionist.
- ☑ Using words like "never again" and "always" in the rule will never work for me.
- ☑ Using this method will strip me of my food choices / sense of autonomy with food.

You'll soon see these notions are all unfounded. Let's address them one by one.

YOU DON'T NEED TO USE THE WORD "PIG" IF IT BOTHERS YOU

Gaining more control of your eating *increases* self-esteem regardless of what you call your lower self. "Pig" was a moniker that worked well *for me.* You can use something different if you prefer. In fact, it's often helpful to customize the term for your lower self to your personal needs.

The "Pig" concept is a big part of my back story. It caught on like wildfire. You'll hear it in hundreds of podcasts, radio shows, coaching demonstrations, and other guest appearances, and see it referenced in forums and discussion groups across the internet. At a minimum, I wanted you to know it so you could make use of these very illustrative, free resources. *(Get them via the free readers' community on www.DefeatYourCravings.com.)*

Alternative monikers work just as well as "Pig," provided you don't pick a name that makes you want to nurture your lower self like an inner wounded child, i.e., "Kitty Cat." This is a game of ruthless domination, not loving yourself thin. I know many people initially cringe at this, so please hear me out before you decide.

You see, at the moment of temptation, when every bone in your body is screaming for a donut, you'll need a strong, primitive reaction to stop the train in its tracks; you'll need a name that makes you wake up and say, *"Whoa! Wait a minute! Who's in charge here?"* One that reminds you there's a real threat to everything important to you. One that might make you feel sick to your stomach, so it *forces* you to pay attention and take back the reins.

Anything that fosters this reaction is fine. Terms such as "Pig," "Food Monster," "Eating Machine," etc., are all good options. It's up to you what you choose to use. But whatever you call it, please know this destructive part of you doesn't care one bit if giving in to your cravings destroys all your hopes dreams, nor how much it hurts you *(or your loved ones)* to get its junk.

If you do move away from "Pig," you'll want to change the rest of the metaphor too. For example, if your *Pig* doesn't *Squeal for Slop*, maybe your *Creature Cries for Crud*? Or perhaps your *Monster Moans for Mush*? Does your *Screecher Scream for Scraps*? It's up to you, just be consistent.

Lastly, some people believe separating from their lower self prevents them from loving themselves completely. This is an overextension of the Gestalt and Jungian concepts of embracing all disowned parts of our identity *(e.g., our "shadow")* to achieve mental well-being. The Pig is a wholly different concept. It's not part of your identity any more than your bladder is. It doesn't deserve to be elevated to human status. It's just a "thing" which generates biological urges that *interfere* with your ability to act on your own best judgment. If you foster love for it, it will take over and run the show! Alpha-wolf style domination is required.

For example, I need to pee right now, but I'm in the middle of writing this important section. I'll lose momentum if I let my bladder interrupt, so it'll just have to wait. My ability to separate my human goals from this biological urge allows me to make progress on my dreams. My bladder isn't in charge; I am. That *contributes* to my mental well-being; it doesn't detract from it. Of course, I must always take care of my biological needs within reason. I can't wait forever, or my body *will* take over. The point is, I have the capacity to delay and choose when and how to express my biological urges. This is a big part of what makes me human.

I'm not by any means arguing against nurturing your inner wounded child or doing "shadow work." These are indeed valuable pursuits. But don't confuse the process of emotional healing with the very practical steps necessary to take control of food. Defeating your cravings means using your intellect to make important food choices, not allowing them to be dictated by whims, emotions, and impulses.

After working with thousands of people, I've developed the impression that those who focus on accepting and expressing their feelings to overcome overeating don't make much progress. Naming the lower self in a way that engenders love and nurturing unfortunately isn't very effective at defeating food cravings.

For this reason, I recommend aggressively separating your "Pig" from your higher self no matter what name you choose. The "Pig," your lower self by definition, *only* wants you to act against your own best judgment. There's nothing lovable about this, so name it accordingly.

AREN'T FOOD RULES DANGEROUS? DON'T THEY CAUSE CRAVINGS?

Rules work better than guidelines because they require less willpower.

"Eat healthy 90% of the time but indulge 10%" is some very common advice, but when, specifically, does the 10% apply? As logical as this advice might seem on

the surface, it provides no actual decision-making guidance. This leaves you to make difficult food choices all day long, which is problematic since research suggests willpower is like a tank of "decision-making gas" – it's full when you wake up but burned up throughout the day. After enough decisions, the tank runs low, and you must rest and refuel or else risk making unhealthy mistakes.

Rules preserve willpower by making difficult food decisions for you ahead of time. *"I'll never again eat chocolate on a weekday,"* worked much better for me than, *"I avoid chocolate 90% of the time,"* because it eliminated all my weekday chocolate decisions. Starbucks on a Wednesday was no longer a grueling, decision-making, willpower-burning experience.

Before adopting crystal-clear rules, when I was just "trying to eat less chocolate," I was unknowingly exhausting my willpower. After adopting my rules, it was much easier to make the right choice. Plus, knowing the *exact* location of the bullseye made me more aware of when I was about to miss it! Apparently, my grandfather was right when he said, "If you don't know what you're aiming at, you'll probably hit something else." *(Apparently this is a variation on Yogi Berra's theme, "If you don't know where you're going, you might wind up somewhere else.")*

The point is soft guidelines require too much decision making. Replacing them with hard and fast rules eliminates this willpower-fatiguing situation. Use rules to regulate your most difficult cravings and save your willpower for more important things!

The next major objection to food rules comes from the mindful-eating community. They argue that rules are a type of dangerous mental restriction that stimulates rebellious feelings which "make" you binge. Accordingly, these people are against anything that separates good versus bad foods. "Food is just food," they say and suggest you "allow" all of it.

In one way, they're right. Rules do indeed stimulate rebellious feelings. The moment you create one, a part of you wants to break it. But I strongly disagree that we should fear this! Rebellion is just one of many emotions with the capacity to stimulate cravings. Emotions are not to be feared, but rather subjugated to our intellect where important decisions are concerned. Feelings aren't facts. Why treat them like as such?

Plus, it's a very short-sighted view of human nature to suggest it's impossible to experience feelings without acting on them. This includes rebellious feelings. Make important food decisions with your head, don't worship your feelings at all costs. Why am I the only one saying this?

More importantly, I've run into hundreds of people using the mindful approach with some success who nevertheless complain they're unable eat as healthfully as they'd like. It's the price they pay for relying entirely on mindful eating to guide them.

The problem is, in a world where it's legal to use unimaginable chemicals and still label the product "food," the line must be drawn somewhere. At some point you need to stand up and say, *"No! That's not food; at least not for me!"*

This is why I prefer to adopt clear rules defining how I want to eat, then manage whatever my rebellious inner two-year-old throws at me.

Now please understand, I do believe in trying to eat more mindfully. People eat less and absorb more nutrition when they do. The problem is, we don't live in a world where it's possible to be mindful all the time. Screaming kids, the boss' demands, last-minute meetings, deadlines, family events, traffic on the road, etc., constantly impinge on our ability to peacefully experience the present moment. So, we need rules to protect us when it's not possible to eat mindfully in much the same way we need rules of the road to protect us when we can't drive mindfully. In a perfect world, everyone would be exquisitely present, alert, and calm enough to avoid accidents. Nevertheless, I'm pretty sure removing all traffic lights in NYC and just encouraging people to drive mindfully would be a recipe for disaster.

So, are food rules dangerous? In my opinion, they are much the opposite. I see them as promoting discipline, confidence, healthy eating, and self-esteem. However, it *is* possible to use them to support over-restriction and undernourishment. If you cut calories or nutrition to such a degree that you're not meeting your authentic biological needs, the Squeals will become louder, seem more appealing, and your body will want to force you to be less discriminating with food. In other words, it will be much more difficult to make healthy choices.

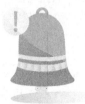

Strongly advise against using rules to over-restrict caloric and nutritional intake.

It's better to focus on easy-to-follow rules that eliminate overeating and give you a sense of confidence and control. After that, you can drop *some* caloric intake to lose weight. Think of a food rule like a sharp kitchen knife – *you can use it to chop vegetables or for more destructive purposes.* Chop vegetables!

WARNING

If you engage in purging behavior and/or have drastically reduced calories and/or nutrition beyond safe levels in the past, then you'll need to be more cautious with eating rules. You can still use the method, but the direct supervision of a licensed medical professional is required so you don't fall into dangerous over-restriction practices. Even if you haven't done this previously, stay alert to the possibility you might be over restricting if you begin losing weight too quickly *(more than a pound or two per week)* and/or if you find yourself ravenously hungry a good portion of the time.

Enough said. Let's talk about the next major objection to adopting crystal clear food rules, the fear of perfectionism.

SHOULDN'T YOU STRIVE FOR PROGRESS, NOT PERFECTION?

Many people fear rules are too perfectionistic, and therefore set them up for failure. "Progress, not perfection" in the mantra they think of when they first encounter the idea. But this reflects a serious misunderstanding of the *constructive* energy in perfectionism. With the distinction between higher versus lower self in place, you can leverage this energy.

The problem with "progress not perfection" when dealing with powerful cravings is that all it really means is *"I'll try for a little while until I don't feel like it anymore!"* The Pig will use this to wear you down. *"Have you tried long enough yet? Is now a good time yet to eat some Slop? You can't be perfect you know. How about now? C'mon, you're going to give in eventually!"* This constant chatter creates doubt and insecurity, wastes mental energy, and makes it harder to focus on the goal.

Winning archers commit with perfection. They don't let go of the arrow until they can see and feel it hitting the bullseye. This lets them focus all their energy on the target, which makes success more likely. So, too, it is with food. You must allow no room for the psychological cancers of doubt and insecurity as you take aim. Rather, you must confidently commit with perfection.

I know what you're thinking. *"If I say I'm 'never' going to do XYZ again and I mess up, I'm going to feel guilty and beat myself up. I've got enough guilt, shame, and negative thinking in my life, thank you very much. Plus, everyone misses their target sometimes, even professional archers! So, I can't aim with perfection, I just can't."*

Not so fast!

When an archer misses the bullseye, they assess how far off the mark they were, in what direction, and then make the necessary adjustments. They soak up all the information they can from every single shot to do better the next time. They don't say *"OMG, I'm a pathetic archer! I might as well just give up and shoot the rest of the arrows up into the air."*

> **Successful archers commit with perfection but forgive themselves with dignity.**

This makes the most of the natural trial-and-error learning mechanism in the brain.

> **When you aim, perfectly commit to your target. When you make a mistake, switch to the "progress not perfection" mindset and learn all you can.**

Most people do the exact opposite when it comes to food. They think "progress not perfection" or *"I'll just do the best I can,"* as they aim, which means they'll try for a little while, screw up, then ruthlessly attack themselves until they feel too weak to resist indulging again. In turn, this prevents learning and builds the *illusion* of powerlessness and hopelessness, which increases the odds of eating *more* Slop. They get stuck in this cycle because, despite the long-term pain. Slop is a very yummy short-term reward which reinforces this line of thinking.

Winners of any sport, business, or game of life commit with perfection and forgive themselves with dignity.

Now, guilt does serve a purpose, just as physical pain does. Without physical pain you wouldn't know when you touched a hot stove or ran into a sharp edge. Pain is an essential attention-getting mechanism.

That said, once you realize you've touched a hot stove, it's best to tend to the wound, make note of how to avoid it; and then let go of the experience. You're not supposed to say *"OMG! I'm a pathetic hot stove toucher! I might as well just put my whole hand down on it."*

Getting stuck on guilt for a food mistake after you've made the necessary adjustments only serves to wear you down and makes it more likely you'll overindulge again. One way to let go of the excessive guilt is to collect evidence of *success* instead of *failure*. Had five cupcakes instead of fifteen? Great! Ate too much at the restaurant but stopped afterwards? Fantastic! Finished off a whole pizza? At least you didn't eat the box!

I'm only half kidding.

The questions you ask yourself determine the evidence you collect, and the evidence you collect determines the identity you build. Asking *"What did I do right?"* and *"How can I stop overeating?"* is infinitely better than asking *"What's wrong with me?"* and *"Why can't I stop?"* Keep asking yourself *"Why can't I stop overeating?"* and you'll actually be instructing your brain to find evidence that you can't. Collect enough proof that you're "powerless" and you'll start to believe it. But collect evidence that you *can* stop, and you'll begin to believe that too.

It's not rocket science, but most people do the exact wrong thing.

Okay, let's move on to common objections to the wording of food rules.

FEAR OF THE WORDS NEVER AND ALWAYS

I always insist on including the words "never" and/or "always" because rules that don't contain these words are just guidelines, not statements of personal law. There's nothing wrong with guidelines as a kind of "north star" to point you in the right direction, but they have built-in loopholes. Without "never again" and/or "always," the guidelines created are much too squishy and non-committal.

For example, one person might say, *"I try to avoid chocolate on weekdays,"* while another states *"I will never again eat chocolate on a weekday."* Who do you think is more likely to eat a piece of chocolate on a Wednesday afternoon?

"Never" and "always" are the only words that can truly nail down a food rule. Anything else creates a loophole the Pig can barrel through. If you "avoid chocolate on weekdays," your Pig will keep saying that you've been doing a pretty good job avoiding it so why not indulge now? You'll have to keep making chocolate decisions, become exhausted, and become much more likely to give in to the craving.

"Never" and "Always" rules are statements of character.

Character is nothing more than what you habitually do at the moment of temptation. Articulating this gives you the power to become the kind of person with food you've always wanted to be with food. Moreover, character trumps willpower, and rules-based character building is a natural process everyone engages in all the time without even knowing!

For example, suppose the elderly lady in front of you in line at the grocery store dropped a ten-dollar bill without realizing it. Nobody else is around to witness this. There's nobody behind you and no video camera recording the scene. Nobody would see you take the money. Do you pick up the money and secretly stash it away for yourself?

When asked this very question, most people reflexively say, "No!"

"Why not?" I ask.

"Because I'm not a thief," they say.

"Doesn't it take a lot of willpower to resist?"

"No!"

"Why not?"

"It's not even an option because I'm not a thief! I never steal!"

And that's the point. It takes no willpower because character trumps willpower.

Moreover, everyone, by virtue of having been raised in a civil society, has naturally encoded *unwritten* character rules in place. For example, as a matter of character, I'll bet you never push people over in the street, kick policemen in the tush, or go #2 in your mother-in-law's living room. Even when there's no chance of getting caught, it's just not the kind of person you are.

Adding more character rules about food to your arsenal is easy. If you have a brain, you're naturally built for it. Biologically speaking, character functions as a kind of behavioral shortcut to preserve energy for more important things. Character minimizes the amount of decision making by pre-making choices for us. And rules build character.

WHAT IF I NEED TO CHANGE MY FOOD RULE LATER ON?

Next, people rightly anticipate needing to change their "never again" or "always" rules later. Experience, consultations with experts, emerging nutritional research, and/or changing health conditions may require modifications down the road, so, they reason it would be foolish to cement their rules in stone.

But the thing is, I'm only suggesting you present things *to the Pig* as if they were set in stone because it's too immature *(and potentially risky)* to entertain anything else! When my little niece was two, I told her she could never cross the road without holding my hand. *"Never ever, ever,"* I said! I knew we'd teach her to look both ways so she could cross the street by herself when she got older, so, why did I lie? Because a two-year-old isn't mature enough to even *think* about crossing the road on her own. I didn't even want the image in her head because it could motivate her to dart out into the street. It was too dangerous. So, I lied and said, *"Never,"* not *"I'll teach you when you're a big girl."*

So, always present food rules to the Pig as if they were set in stone, which require either the "never again" or "always" words.

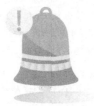

Despite this, you can change your food plan anytime with forethought and consideration.

(A food plan is how I refer to your full set of food rules.)

To change your food plan, first save a copy, then write down what you want to change and why. If you still think it's a good idea, go ahead and make the change. But allow 24 hours before it goes into effect! This way you'll know it's *you* who is making the change, not the Pig.

You don't need to fear getting "boxed in forever" by food rules. They're just how you draw a boundary around the bullseye so you can aim with precision and learn from mistakes. Without this feedback, you can't hope to improve.

HOW CAN YOU POSSIBLY KNOW WHAT YOU'LL NEVER DO AGAIN? OR WHAT YOU WILL ALWAYS DO WITHOUT FAIL?

The next objection to the words "never" and "always" is that nobody can know what will happen in the future, so it's dishonest to commit. Besides, what if you forget?

Thought experiment: A man says to his fiancée, "I really *want* to never sleep with another women, but I can't predict the future and there sure are a lot of attractive people out there! Besides, what if I forget?"

There are some promises we're expected to make with certainty. Either you plan to remember, or you plan to forget. Making 100% commitments is a part of life. Otherwise, you might become a confirmed bachelor *(or bachelorette)*.

As a practical matter, many people do forget their rules during the learning process. That's why, in Defeat Your Cravings, the "consciously and purposefully" clause is assumed to be implicitly appended to every food rule. When I say, *"I will never again eat chocolate during the week,"* what I really mean is, *"I will never again consciously and purposefully eat chocolate during the week."* This way, if I happen to eat some by accident, I'll stop the moment I realize it, knowing I haven't broken my rule. If I continued to eat more, however, then I would've broken my promise.

WON'T FOOD RULES DEPRIVE ME OF THE FREEDOM TO EAT WHAT I LOVE?

Geneen Roth first pointed out that nobody ever really chooses between deprivation and indulgence, but rather between two different types of deprivation: The kind you feel when you don't indulge versus the kind you feel when you do.

For example, if I never eat chocolate again, I'll forever deprive myself of the feel, taste, and texture of chocolate. I'll also never again get "high" from all the sugar, fat, caffeine, and theobromine in chocolate. On the other hand, if I keep eating it, I'll be depriving myself of being a tall, thin man who walks in the world with confidence and strength. I'll lose the peace of mind that comes from being free of worry about cardiovascular disease, diabetes, and other diet-preventable or reversible conditions. I'll be unnecessarily burdened by cravings and the "Pig" will continue to bother me with incessant excuses to indulge.

The "Pig" says I can either indulge and feel good or abstain and feel deprived. It's not that simple though, because to indulge I must sacrifice—*to at least some extent*—important goals and dreams. See, there are *two* types of deprivation, and you're always choosing between them. Most people never consider what they give up by *not* depriving themselves of immediate food pleasure.

Lastly, every time you indulge a craving, you deprive yourself of the opportunity to weaken it because the only way to defeat the actual craving is to deny it. The only way out is through, and every craving is an opportunity for self-love versus self-harm. *(Much more on the cravings extinction process later.)*

Finally, stop overstimulating your taste buds with hyper-palatable, concentrated forms of sugar, starch, fat, salt, and excitotoxins, and they'll double in sensitivity after just a few months. That means while you may not find foods in their natural state enjoyable right now, in just a few months they'll taste significantly more delicious to you! The impact of this phenomenon is greater the less processed food you consume.

This is due to processes called "downregulation" and "upregulation."

I first experienced downregulation when I lived close to a subway overpass in NYC. At first, the noise was so loud I couldn't sleep, but a month later I had no trouble falling asleep because my nervous system stopped responding as strongly after it was overstimulated for a while.

The same thing happens if you eat a chocolate bar every day. The first time it tastes like heaven. The second time, a little less so. The third, even less. After a few months, it's hardly pleasurable at all. In fact, it may just seem like you need chocolate to feel "normal," and it may even become difficult to derive pleasure from natural foods. This is why so many people say they hate fruits and vegetables. Even though humans evolved to love them, our senses have been blunted by overprocessed, industrial food.

Thankfully, the nervous system also *upregulates* when you remove or moderate the offenders. It only takes a few months to notice this difference.

I'd like to postulate a strong reason why human taste buds are so prone to change their preferences: In primitive times, when food sources were scarce or constantly shifting, it was dangerous to get "stuck" on any one food because we might've starved. We needed to crave whatever happened to be available. Today, you can teach your brain what's "available" by skillfully crafting food rules, and your taste buds will learn to like what *is* available.

So, the first answer to the idea that food rules will take away the freedom to eat what you love is, what you love will change and you'll likely get *more* pleasure from food, not less. You don't need to believe me you only have to try it.

But the second part of the answer to the fear that food discipline will reduce your freedom is that exactly the opposite is usually the case! Every time you add discipline to your life you're expanding your freedom, not restricting it. For example, a jazz pianist acquires freedom to express her soul *only* after practicing the structure and discipline of music for years. Without this, the music wouldn't "hold together" underneath her creative expression. Similarly, the discipline of the engineers who built your car is what makes it possible for your tires to turn the exact amount required when you rotate the steering wheel. This gives you the freedom to drive and expands your radius of locomotion!

Bottom line, if you're concerned the discipline of a new food rule will deprive you, try focusing not only on what you'll deprive yourself of if you adopt it, but also what you'll deprive yourself of if you don't. A well-informed choice always favors you no matter which way you go, so there's never any harm in comparing. Most people tend to just consider what they'll be missing out on in the near term if they adopt a food rule, not what indulging in the craving will deprive them of in the future.

I'll exit this chapter with a powerful story which puts this in perspective. When I was about forty, toward the end of my most serious food struggles, I lived in New Hampshire. Once a week I'd drive up to the White Mountains for a hike. My favorite activity was tackling a 5,000+ foot mountain with a ton of junk food *(mostly chocolate, sugary granola, potato chips, etc.)* in tow. I'd enthusiastically snack on this before, during, and after the hike. My Pig had me convinced a hike wasn't a hike without it. As far as it was concerned, Slop was survival gear as important as my headlamp or compass.

One day I realized I didn't know what it was like to hike *without* junk food. I'd simply never done it, not even once, and wondered what I might be missing. So instead of the traditional bags, boxes, bars, and containers, I packed up some organic greens, blueberries, a thermos full of green tea, and some seeds. As I walked the trail an incredible calmness came over me – *something I didn't know anyone could feel.* It was like I was breathing the air for the first time, hearing the running water, and appreciating the sites like never before. I thoroughly enjoyed every animal I encountered. It was one of the best days of my life!

I was left with a feeling of "rightness" in the world, which, ever since then, has been a more powerful lure than any craving. This lasted several days. I slept better and felt less reactive to "emergencies." I was better with my clients. I solved problems easily and more effectively. In many ways I was more present than I'd ever been.

Through this experience, I realized that by refusing to deprive myself of Slop, I'd actually been depriving myself of who I was genuinely meant to be. My Pig wanted me to think hiking without Slop was a cruel and torturous deprivation. It turns out I'd been so distracted by the delicious tastes I had no idea that I was, in fact, *truly* depriving myself.

I've since learned this experience of *contentment* is available just below the surface to anyone who wants it, but sadly, most let their Pig keep it from them. This upsets me to no end.

Now, if you think I'm suggesting you hug trees and avoid certain foods, you're missing the point. The point is, there are *two* types of deprivation and you're always free to choose. When the Pig says, *"You can't follow these food rules any longer, they're too depriving,"* pause to ask yourself what it will deprive *you* of if you break them.

> *"The flame that burns twice as bright, burns half as long."*
>
> Lao Tzu

With these objections to a rules-based approach debunked, we can proceed to helping you choose your first simple rule!

START WITH ONE SIMPLE RULE

Imagine one stroke of a pen changing your life. This is not a fantasy. It can and does happen all the time. The clarity, commitment, and confidence your first rule provides you with makes all the difference.

Most people try way too hard to defeat their cravings. In these cases, the Pig's favorite game is setting the bar too high, so they'll eventually give in. Slowly turning the ship around and letting go of the diet mentality works better. This means pushing aside weight loss for at least a few weeks until a sense of power over your cravings is restored. Of course, this assumes a doctor hasn't instructed you otherwise.

The diet mentality says you must be as strict as possible and lose weight as quickly as possible until you reach your goal. Then, the theory goes, you can go back to eating "normally." But this almost never pans out. Dieting signals to the brain it's living in an environment of scarce calories and nutrition, which makes food feel like an urgent need. When the diet is "over" and calories are once again available, the brain wants to hoard as much food as possible. This would be a good strategy for survival if you lived in a feast-or-famine environment 100,000 years ago, but it's a horrific approach in the modern food environment.

There is evidence which suggests that dieting to lose weight may be associated with increased risk of future obesity and weight gain. For example, Siahpush et al. (2015) reported on a study with 8,824 people in the *International Journal of Behavioral Medicine* which found that, "...compared to those who were never on a diet in the previous year, the odds of obesity were 1.9, 2.9, and 3.2 times higher among those who were on a diet once, more than once, and always, respectively."

Juhaeri et al. (2004) also published a study with 10,554 people in the *European Journal of Epidemiology,* which suggested that self-reported dieting was associated with a larger average annual weight gain than non-dieting over a period of six years.

And a five-year, longitudinal study of 2,516 people published in the *Journal of the American Dietetic Association* concluded that, "...dieting may lead to weight gain via the long-term adoption of behavioral patterns counterproductive to weight management." (Neumark⊠Sztainer et al. 2007)

While there is also evidence to the contrary *(that dieting will not lead to individuals overeating in the future)* the studies I've cited are extraordinarily consistent with what my team and I have witnessed working with almost 2,000 clients over the past eight years. So instead of rushing to lose weight by over-restricting and dieting, the *Defeat Your Cravings* method suggests moving the needle in the right direction in a sustainable, enjoyable way. Like my grandfather used to say, *"You've got to go to kindergarten before you can go to college."*

Now, if you already have rules that work for you, you don't need to change them. After all, *"If it ain't broke, don't fix it!"* That's something else my grandpa used to say. He said a lot of things.

Also, if you *really* need more than one rule to protect yourself from dangerous overeating at the outset, then go ahead and add more. But the overarching principle still holds: start as simply as you can, protect yourself, and don't overcomplicate or over-restrict. Make it so easy to get started that you'll have no trouble complying even when your motivation is on the floor. The momentum you'll gain from observing yourself consistently doing something *(anything)* constructive with food is required for the rest of the journey.

Here are some key points to remember:

- ☑ Nobody will tell you what to eat.
- ☑ Your rule is entirely up to you.
- ☑ You can change your rule any time with forethought and consideration.
- ☑ Don't allow your Pig to make you feel too guilty for mistakes.
- ☑ You'll present the rule to the Pig as if it's set in stone, but you and I know you'll probably tweak it down the road.

With this understanding, there's no reason not to get started right away.

HOW TO CHOOSE ONE SIMPLE RULE

Choose something you can and will do, which does not create a dramatic caloric or nutritional deficit and is something you can easily sustain. If your rule is too restrictive, your brain will force you to be less discriminating with food, and the Pig will seem more persuasive. Starting with something both simple and sustainable stops the biological imperatives that make you want to give in and/or "consume mass quantities."

Expect to experiment with this first rule for a week or two before reassessing it. Consider this a starting point. Your first rule may work wonders, but it may need tweaking, so just pick something you can live with.

To start, ask yourself:

> **"What's the simplest, easiest rule which would make a big difference, but also not be too burdensome, depriving, or restrictive?"**

Pause for a moment to see what comes to mind before you read the examples below. You'll notice no matter what rule you consider the Pig will say you can't do it. It'll scream that you've failed a million times before and try to convince you that this time will be no different. But remember, even if you've been driving on a highway for 1,000 miles, you can still take the next exit. Don't give in.

As you consider adopting the first rule, the Pig may focus on your last indulgence as evidence that sticking to this rule will be impossible. But it doesn't matter if you overate five seconds ago or have a whole box of cookies in your mouth right now. Simply see what comes to mind in response to the question above and write down a few guesses. Remember this isn't a school room and there are no right or wrong answers. Think of it more like a game where you're inventing rules which *might* work. So, what rules come to mind for you?

Examples of successful rules include:

☑ **Adding Healthy Behaviors**

- I'll always drink 16 ounces of purified water before each meal.
- I'll always walk ten full minutes before sitting down at my computer every day.
- I'll never go to sleep at night without writing down a hypothetical food plan for the next day.

☑ **Moderation and Portion Control**

- I'll never again eat more than two servings of pasta per calendar week.
- I'll never go back for seconds again.
- I'll never eat more than three meals and one snack per calendar day again, and there will always be at least two hours between the end of each meal or snack and the beginning of the next one.

☑ **Eliminating Unhealthy Foods**

- I'll never eat anything sweet again besides whole fruit, berries, and stevia.
- I'll never buy food at a ballpark again.
- I'll never eat fried food again.

☑ **Eliminating Unwanted Food Behaviors**

- I'll never again eat in front of a screen.
- I'll never eat while driving again.
- I'll never again eat while standing up and cooking.
- I'll always put my fork down between bites.

Close your eyes and ask the question again:

"What's the simplest, easiest rule which would make a big difference, but also not be too burdensome, depriving, or restrictive?"

Dare to push beyond the inevitable, "I don't know." If you don't know, nobody does. But you *do* know. You do, you do, you do! Dare to be wrong and write it down. Then ask these final questions to be sure the rule is rock solid.

Does your food rule include the words "never again" or "always?" If it doesn't, your Pig will think you don't mean business, as previously discussed.

Does it overly restrict calories or nutrition? The intent of the first rule is only to give you more control and confidence during this initial implementation phase. You can adjust for weight loss in a week or two.

Lastly, remember, you're not making the commitment yet, so just take your best guess. Your first intuition is usually the right choice.

TYPES OF RULES

There are four categories of food rules to consider:

☑ **Never Rules:** What will you *never* indulge in again? Foods, drinks, and behaviors. For example, *"I will never again eat chocolate."*

☑ **Always Rules:** What will you *always* do regarding food, drinks, and eating behavior? Perhaps you always start your day with five ounces of leafy green vegetables in a smoothie with 300 calories of fruit and berries. Maybe you always take a picture of your meal before you eat it. *(This heightens awareness and works for many people.)*

☑ **Conditional Rules:** What will you permit only in certain amounts, at certain times, and/or under certain conditions? Unambiguously specify these conditions so you'll know when the light is red versus green. In your Pig's way of thinking, a yellow light is really green, so there can be no "maybe" in a food rule. An example of a conditional rule is: *"I will never again eat pretzels except at a ballgame."*

☑ **Unrestricted:** What foods and/or behaviors will you permit without restriction? For example, *"I may eat as many unsauced leafy-green vegetables as I like at any time."*

THE ACID TEST FOR YOUR RULE

The Pig barrels through ambiguity like a race car driver at the Grand Prix on crack. Leaving little things undefined creates rips in the fabric of your rule which the Pig will tug at it until the rule no longer means anything.

For example, *"I will never again eat sugar more than once per week,"* sounds like a good rule, but what is sugar? Can you have whole fruit? What about the sweeteners in commercial spaghetti sauce? Ketchup? Honey in your tea? Artificial sweeteners? There's too much ambiguity for the rule to hold. So, try to be more specific. You could rephrase the rule to state *"Except for one serving of dessert per calendar week, I will never again consume any sweet taste besides whole fruit, berries, and stevia."* With sugar and starch, I've found it's best to list what you *can* eat, not what you *can't*. Lengthen the list as necessary.

The acid test for every rule is: **Could ten outside observers totally agree about whether you followed your rule or not if they followed you around for a month?** The answer for the first sugar rule above is clearly "no" because the definition of "sugar" leaves too much room for interpretation. Only the second answer passes the test.

Take some time to eliminate ambiguity from your rule until it passes the test.

VACATIONS, RESTAURANTS, FAMILY AND SOCIAL EVENTS TRAVEL, AND OTHER EXCEPTIONS

You can adjust your food rules for vacations, family and social events, restaurants, travel, holidays, and other exceptions, provided you're specific about the boundaries. For example, *"The only sweet taste I will ever consume again is whole fruit except for Thanksgiving, Christmas, and New Year's, when I may have one serving of any dessert of my choosing."* Or maybe you never eat bread except for two pieces at a restaurant each week. It's up to you.

The point is you can make exceptions to your day-to-day rules by specifying the conditions and boundaries. This gives you tremendous flexibility. However, there are two caveats.

First, the boundaries you instill must be clear, so you won't need willpower to know when to stop. It's like drawing additional rings on your archery target. You shoot for the bullseye every day but widen the target for well-specified special occasions. Each ring has a clear boundary just like the bullseye, for all the same reasons. This is particularly important when planning for rare treats because the brain releases extra dopamine when it encounters a rich source of calories outside its ordinary routine. Exceptions are extra pleasurable for this reason, so you'll want more. Make sure your boundaries are set up in a way that it's 100% clear to you when to stop.

Here's the second caveat: not everyone can successfully moderate their treats using conditional rules. Some need to abstain entirely. The ability to moderate is also specific to each treat. For example, someone who must abstain from sugar might still be able to moderate flour, chips, or nuts, etc. This is mostly determined by trial and error. However, if you've made four or more attempts to moderate a given food with conditional rules and it's still not working, you should probably abstain. For a more detailed worksheet to help make these decisions, download the free reader bonuses at www.DefeatYourCravings.com

Lastly, there's always risk involved with conditional rule experiments. It's difficult to determine who can and who can't moderate hyper-palatable foods ahead of time; so, you'll need to decide for yourself if the freedom to indulge is worth the risk of overeating. I can't take that risk *for* you.

Do you want to add any rings to your archery target by adding clearly defined, conditional exceptions to your simple rule *(or rules)?*

DON'T GET TOO RESTRICTIVE

Does your rule allow for regular, reliable nutrition without becoming too hungry?

I've seen approximately double the success rate for those who focus on regular, reliable nutrition versus trying to lose weight too quickly. So even though every bone in your body might be screaming for a rule to help you lose weight fast, please at least consider the possibility that slow and steady wins the race.

Then modify your rule as necessary.

YOU ARE 100% FREE TO DECIDE WHAT YOU EAT

In the end, nobody is going to follow you around all day, see what food you buy, take out of the containers, put in your mouth, chew, and swallow; so, nobody can decide what's the best rule for you but you. Read books and consult with experts, but also understand that dependency is a core problem in overeating. Ultimately, *autonomous responsibility is required* to defeat your cravings. This involves a fundamental decision to become the master of your own destiny.

COMMIT

Put your hand over your heart, take a deep, long breath in, and an even longer breath out. Then read your rule out loud. Then say: *"I commit to following this rule 100% no matter what my Pig says to the contrary."* With at least one simple rule *(or simple set of rules)* in hand, you're ready to start disempowering the cancerous logic behind your Pig's Squeals!

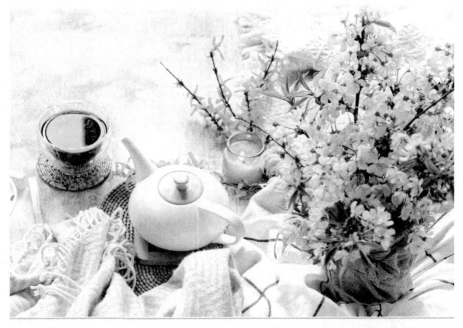

ELIMINATE YOUR ENEMY'S EXCUSES

The clarity of "One Simple Rule" heightened my awareness of my reptilian brain. With my rules in place, I could more easily tell when that part of my brain was being activated. The rule created a reliable space between stimulus and response which made it possible to experiment with a host of other techniques too. The earliest and most important of these was tearing down the false logic in the Pig's excuses.

The first Squeal I attacked was the one about "emotional eating." The Pig had long convinced me that overeating was caused by emotional trauma. It would repeatedly tell me this because it knew it would take years to fully heal and, in the meantime, it could keep eating Slop.

The Pig said my emotions were like a fire that had to be extinguished before I could make any progress with food. After my "awakening," however, I realized

I didn't need to put out the fire, only to stop the Pig from poking holes in the fireplace.

Sticking with this analogy, a roaring fire in a well-contained fireplace is an *asset*, not a liability. People gather round, tell stories, hug, cry, laugh, and make memories. It is only when ashes escape that the fire can do any damage. But the Pig was a master at poking holes in the fireplace with its false logic!

The mantra "fix the fireplace, not the fire" became my new motto. Don't get bogged down solving emotional trauma. Instead, identify the logical problems with the Pig's excuses to indulge. This made a tremendous difference.

I still believe it's helpful to work on emotional conflict. In fact, I rather enjoy that kind of work. But these days it's not my primary focus, because you can defeat your cravings in a month or two with simple techniques that require no soul searching at all.

Therefore, our goal is to sever the link between emotions and overeating, not to psychoanalyze ourselves to heal all our emotional pain. At this point, after working with approximately 2,000 clients, I'm convinced this is a *critical* shift in mindset. I've observed less than half the success rate among those who insisted on doing the emotional work first as compared to those who embrace the idea of severing the link between emotions and overeating.

Now, I didn't personally have all the tools in this book while I was recovering. I defeated my cravings almost entirely through a personal cravings and Squeals journal that I kept for about eight years before publishing. Basically, whenever I made a mistake, I made it a priority to analyze what was wrong with the Pig's excuses that had preceded the episode. I just kept asking: **"How did my Pig lie to me to get me to feed it Slop?"** and **"How was its argument based on a lie?"**

For example, the Pig often tricked me as follows: *"Hey, Bubba,* (this is what the Pig calls me sometimes), *you can't keep up this level of vigilance forever, it's exhausting! Eventually you'll get fatigued, drop your guard, and I'll get you then! So, you might as well just get it over with and feed me. Omnonmnomnom! Yippee!! C'mon, you know you want to. Please?"*

At first this was very difficult for me to refute because, on the surface, it seemed very appealing. After all, it *is* exhausting to get through the first week of cravings when you change behavior, and it *does* feel like you won't be able to keep at it indefinitely. But eventually I was able to counter with this refutation, *"No, Mr. Pig, I don't have to do this forever, I only need to do it now because the future is an infinite string of present moments; so, if I always eat healthy now, I'll always eat healthy!"* (I was first exposed to the idea that the future is an infinite string of present moments in Jack Trimpey's book *Rational Recovery* (Trimpey 1996)).

A few years later I made it even stronger by adding, *"Pig, you're assuming my 'eat healthy now' muscle will get weaker over time, but muscles get stronger when exercised. Therefore, I only need to keep using my now muscle every day and it'll be stronger in the future, not weaker as you predict! Plus, cravings reduce dramatically when they aren't rewarded, eventually becoming entirely dormant. Besides, you don't have a time machine; so, stop pretending you can see into the future!"*

Can you see how this works?

In the next section I'll show you how to do it yourself. But first, let's recap a few terms introduced above and in the previous chapter which you'll encounter repeatedly as you go forward:

- ☑ **"Reptilian Brain" / "Lizard Brain":** This refers to the brainstem, which appears to be the most primitive part of our neuroanatomy, which is responsible for survival impulses such as fight or flight, mate or ignore, and, most importantly for our purposes, feast or famine. When activated, it can unfortunately override our rational thinking and long-term planning, which is the cause of so much of our troubles with food cravings!

- ☑ **Food Rule:** Any singular rule you create to govern the role you'd like a particular food and/or food behavior to play in your life. For example, *"I will never eat chocolate again except for two ounces on Saturdays,"* or *"I only eat pretzels at major league baseball games,"* or *"I always start my day with a 16-ounce green smoothie before eating anything else."*

- ☑ **Food Plan:** All of your food rules combined, if you have more than one.

☑ **"Pig" or "Inner Pig":** This is a fictional entity which represents your destructive food self – the part of you that wants to use the energy of the reptilian brain to break your rules and indulge cravings you previously swore off indulging. It's our survival drive which has been hijacked by the manufactured food industry into a collection of bad habits. I use it interchangeably with "lower self" in this book.

☑ **"Pig Squeal" or "Squeal":** These are the things the Pig says to get you to break the rules. It's an easy to remember device instead of saying "destructive food thoughts" or "rationalizations and excuses to indulge my cravings." In the example above, the Pig Squeal was: *"Eventually you'll get fatigued, drop your guard, and then I'll get you, so you might as well just indulge your cravings now!"*

☑ **"Refutation":** The logical explanation that proves a Pig Squeal to be wrong. The refutation for the Squeal in the preceding paragraph was: *"The future is an infinite string of present moments; so, if I always eat healthy now, I'll always eat healthy."*

HOW TO ERADICATE ENEMY EXCUSES FOR INDULGENCE

It's a relatively simple matter to refute the Pig's favorite excuses, but it's unfortunately also easy to accept them. Therefore, even if you're good at logical reasoning and this all seems second nature to you, I'd like to request you pay careful attention to this section. My team and I must've reviewed literally more than 10,000 Squeals over the years, and if we learned one thing better than anything else it was this: subtle omissions result in big mistakes! The fireplace metaphor really does hold – allowing even one small hole in the fireplace lets tiny embers escape to burn down the entire house.

Expose the Pig's Soft Underbelly

Suppose your first rule was: *"I'll never again eat after 8 p.m. unless I'm out to dinner."* Any thought, feeling, or impulse which suggests you might eat something at home at 8:01 p.m. or later would qualify as a Squeal. The moment you detect a thought like this one you say, *"Whoa! I see you, Pig!"*

This is called "Separating" and, although it may seem trivial, it's a critical part of the process.

Then say to yourself: *"Go ahead, Pig, tell me why I should break my rules and give in to my craving!"*

Step back and listen for a response.

Maybe your Pig will say something like, *"C'mon, a few bites won't hurt!"* or *"You're so fat a little more won't matter."* Or perhaps, *"Your parents were fat, so you're doomed!"*

Whatever it says, write it down! Don't try to hold it in your head because the limitations of short-term memory will interfere. It feels more natural to just *think* about what's wrong with the Squeal but   writing it down is much more effective.

Sometimes your Pig will have more than one reason to eat Slop. To check for this, ask: *"Why else do you want me to break my rules and give in to my craving?"* Keep asking until there are no more Squeals. Write them all down.

Get the Language Right

Initially you may hear a confusing mixture of "I" versus "you" language in the Squeals. For example: *"My parents were fat, so I'm doomed."*

As silly as it sounds, to fully separate from the Pig, you'll need to change the I's to you's so it's perfectly clear the Squeal belongs to the Pig and not you. *"My parents were fat, so I'm doomed!"* must become *"Your parents were fat, so you're doomed!"* because the Pig is talking *to* you. For simplicity, this is called "Pigifying" the Squeal.

Don't skip clarifying the language.

Separation isn't complete until you do, and without it, the rest of the process won't work.

Expand the Pig's Thoughts

The Pig will try to hide behind an abbreviated version of its Squeal because it knows the full argument won't hold water when exposed to the light of day. Don't let it hide! Expand the Squeal to expose the Pig's soft underbelly – the place in its argument where it's most vulnerable.

Also ask yourself what the Pig might be *implying* in the Squeal. For example, it says: *"Your parents were fat, so you're doomed!"* Well, fat parents couldn't possibly doom a child to a life of obesity unless obesity were largely determined by genetics. So, the Pig's fuller argument is: *"Your parents were fat, and obesity is largely genetic, so you're doomed!"*

The word "doomed" also implies you can't do anything about your fate, so it's not even worth trying. By choosing this word, the Pig is saying obesity is almost *entirely* genetic. Otherwise, you wouldn't be helpless to do anything about it, and it would at least be worth trying. The expanded Squeal is therefore more like: *"Your parents were fat, and obesity is almost entirely genetic. There's little to nothing you can do about it, so it's not even worth trying. You're doomed!"*

Expanding the Pig's logic to include what it's *implying* exposes additional vulnerabilities in its argument.

To finish articulating the Squeal, add what the Pig wants you to do. The Pig always Squeals for a purpose – to get Slop! It wants you to feed it. So, you must add something like, *"Therefore you should break your rules and indulge your cravings now,"* at the end of the Squeal.

This is important because sometimes you can't see a flaw in the Pig's basic argument but only in the idea you should overeat because of what it's saying. You won't see that if you don't add its desired action at the end.

So, the fully expanded example is: *"Your parents were fat, and obesity is almost entirely genetic, so there's little to nothing you can do about it. It's not even worth trying! You're doomed, so you might as well break your rules and indulge your craving now."* If this doesn't quite make sense to you yet, please re-read this last section on expanding the Pig's thoughts.

Expose the Lies and Disempower the Pig's Argument

A Half Truth with a Bigger Lie

The Pig's strategy almost always involves a half-truth coupled with a bigger lie.

The Pig camouflages its faulty argument behind a partial truth, sometimes a strong one, in hopes it will provide enough cover to sneak by your rational brain. For example, *"This ice cream is the most pleasure you can possibly have today, so you simply must eat it!"* The ice cream *may* provide more pleasure than anything else on any given day, but you're capable of abstaining from certain intense, short-term pleasures to pursue more important pleasures longer-term. You can trade the orgasmic pleasure of a chocolate ice cream break on an otherwise difficult day for the knowledge you're moving toward your ideal body, freedom from torturous cravings, more energy, confidence, and a better life overall. It's not at all true that you simply must eat everything that tastes good!

I used to think I had to prove every last one of the Pig's words false. This was exhausting and made me want to give up. Eventually, when I understood its strategy, the refutations became much easier to complete and more effective too. Accept there's some truth in what the Pig says, and you'll be more likely to see the lie and successfully stop the indulgence.

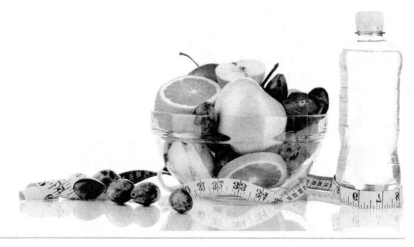

The Three Key Questions to effectively refute the Pig's lies

Once you've fully articulated the Squeal, ask these three critical questions:

01. What's true (or partially true) about what the Pig is saying?

02. Where's the lie (or lies)?

03. What's wrong with its conclusion?

I know I shouldn't break my rules and indulge, but where, specifically, is this Piggy conclusion wrong?

Let's illustrate using the example we've been working on: *"Your parents were fat, so you're doomed!"* Recall this was previously expanded to, *"Your parents were fat, and obesity is almost entirely genetic. There's little to nothing you can do about it, so it's not even worth trying. You're doomed, so you might as well break your rules and indulge your craving now!"*

What's true (or partially true) about this? Genetics does play a significant role in obesity, but on average studies have shown that dietary and lifestyle factors are actually more important. It's an unfortunate fact of life that obese parents make it *more likely* you'll be obese yourself. But it's not a foregone conclusion, it just makes it harder to be thin. My parents were fat, so if I wanted to become a male bikini model, I'd have to work twice as hard as others might. *(No, you can't have the last ten seconds of your life back to get that image of me out of your head.)*

Now, where are the lies? If dietary and lifestyle factors are more important than genetics in driving obesity, it's wildly inaccurate to say it's almost entirely genetic. Genetics may be a factor, but there's a lot more to the story. This means "you can't do anything about it" is clearly false. So, too, is the idea that it's not worth trying, because diet and lifestyle factors are controllable. Even if you couldn't do much about it, does that mean you should do *nothing* and instead try to get as obese as possible? No! Everyone must play the hand they're dealt. So even if everything the Pig said about being genetically doomed to be obese were true, it would *not* follow that you should just break your rules and indulge the cravings!

Create a Short "Hook" to Hold Onto When the Craving Hits

It's important to go through the above process once for each Squeal that bothers you. Save your work and read through it several times during the period you're working on the Squeal. But because you probably won't be able to recall the full refutation the moment a craving hits, you'll also want to create a little "hook" to hold onto. This is a short, pithy statement you can easily recall when you feel most tempted.

Ask yourself which part of the refutation is most powerful. A great refutation should immediately make you feel calmer and in control. So which part provides you with the most relief?

For example, I found it most powerful to recognize diet and lifestyle factors were more important than genetics in determining my obesity outcome, so I created the following mantra: *"My genetics suck but diet and lifestyle are more important!"* That's what I told myself whenever the Pig tried to play the "It's genetic, so you're doomed" card.

In summary, there's the original Squeal where the Pig tries to abbreviate to hide what it's doing. Then there's the Expanded Squeal you get to by thinking about everything the Pig is *implying*.

Next is the full refutation that the comprehensive logical proof that the Pig is lying.

And finally, the Hook is the super-abbreviated refutation you can more easily hold onto in the heat of the moment. *(Periodically review the full refutation until you feel like you don't need to anymore because the Hook easily retrieves the meaning.)*

Let's summarize our work on this Pig Squeal.

SQUEAL: *"Your parents were fat, so you're doomed!"*

EXPANDED SQUEAL: *"Your parents were fat, and obesity is almost entirely genetic. There's little to nothing you can do about it, so it's not even worth trying. You're doomed, so you might as well break your rules and indulge now!"*

FULL REFUTATION: Dietary and lifestyle factors account for more variance in obesity than genetics! Therefore, the idea "you can't do anything about it" is clearly false, as is the idea it's not even worth trying. Even if you could do very little about it, it doesn't mean you should do *nothing* and get as obese as possible.

THE HOOK: *"My genetics may suck but diet and lifestyle are more important!"*

When you're first working on a particular craving you may wish to read your hooks out loud each morning, and the full refutations once or twice per week until the Squeal doesn't bother you anymore.

One more concise example.

PIG SQUEAL: *"You've never stuck with anything before, so why bother now?"*

EXPANDED SQUEAL: *"You've failed to stick to your plans a million times before, so you'll always do so in the future. You never could, so you never will. It's just who you are, so why not just break the rules and indulge your cravings now?"*

FULL REFUTATION: It's true that I've tried dozens of times and failed, but if people couldn't do things they'd never done before we'd all still be crawling around in diapers! Human beings are learning machines. The path to success almost always goes through repeated failure. People who lose weight and keep it off for 5+ years have *more* failed attempts behind them than those who yo-yo up and down. As the old song goes, "With every mistake we must surely be learning." People fall and get up until they stay up. Being on a highway for a thousand miles without taking an exit says nothing about your ability to get off on the next one! The name of the game is staying in the game until you win it.

THE HOOK: *"With every mistake we must surely be learning. The path to success often means experiencing repeated failure."*

SUMMARY OF THE REFUTATION PROCESS

Make a crystal-clear rule. Then wake up when the Pig Squeals to break it. *"I see you, Pig!"* Ask why it wants you to. Write down its answer. Make sure it's in Pig language, using "you" statements not "I" statements. Expand it to include everything the Pig is implying and what it wants you to do. Then ask yourself the following:

01. What's true *(or partially true)* about this?

02. Where are the lies?

03. What's wrong with the Pig's conclusion?

04. Finally, create a short, simple Hook to use when it counts!

Practice whenever you can, since your own refutations will be much more powerful than the ones I suggest. And for the sake of practice, you should even refute the "little" Squeals that don't really tempt you, so you can handle the bigger cravings when they hit.

Above I've illustrated how to refute at the moment of impulse *("real-time refutations")*. However, please know you can also use refutations after mistakes *("postmortem refutations")*. In this case, ask, *"What did the Pig say to get me to break my rules?"*

You can even use the process *proactively* by challenging your Pig each morning, or *(especially)* before you'll be attending a particularly challenging event: *"Okay, Pig, what do you have in store for me today? What's your best reason to get me to break my rules and overeat?"* It's not essential, but it removes the element of surprise for anything the Pig may be planning.

So, there are three ways to use refutations:

01. In real time at the moment of temptation.

02. Post-mortem after mistakes have been made.

03. Proactively.

Now, before I move on to Step 3 in the *Defeat Your Cravings* method, I want to place refutations in context because as powerful as they are, they do have their limitations.

THE LIMITATIONS OF SEPARATION AND REFUTATION

Exposing the false logic in the Pig's argument is like pouring sawdust and glass on the previously greased chute from craving to indulgence. You can still go down it if you want, but it won't be nearly as pleasant because you'll no longer be able to fool yourself into thinking it's okay. This makes it more difficult to overindulge and is at least half the battle.

However, there are limitations to how much separation and refutation can accomplish. While these two steps alone were responsible for the bulk of *my* recovery, I could've done it in months rather than the years it took me if I'd had the tools developed since then. You see, while you can defeat your cravings by just recognizing and refuting the Pig's Squeals, and while for certain cravings you might not need anything else, **there are several additional tools which dramatically enhance, speed, and solidify progress.** Plus, most people experience at least some cravings which don't yield to these two steps alone.

In the next section I'll turn to the first and most important of the additional tools: Disempowering the false sense of emergency underlying most overeating episodes.

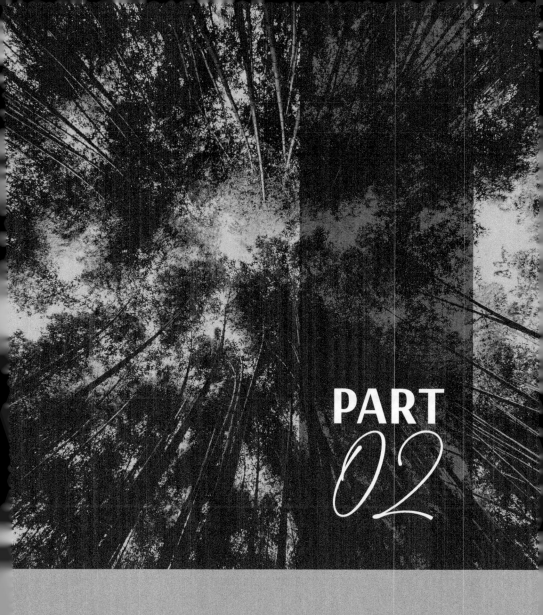

PART
02

ENHANCING AND SPEEDING UP THE PROCESS

TURN OFF THE FALSE ALARMS

About five years ago, a passing comment on a lunch date had an extremely profound impact on my thinking. "Oh, you work with overeaters?" she said. "I used to binge every night before bed, but then I started doing yoga instead. Now I don't binge anymore. *I don't even want to.*"

At the time, I'd practiced some yoga myself but couldn't see the connection. I knew I felt very different at the end of a class but at the time I was only interested in using *thinking* techniques to help with overeating. I was blind to the notion that regulating the nervous system might be important too. In retrospect, this is a big part of why it took me years to recover as compared to the few months it takes successful clients today.

Apparently, the way you breathe in yoga activates the part of the nervous system which allows you to rest, digest, and calmly use your capacity for reason. It's called the parasympathetic nervous system. It takes you out of emergency mode and restores the body and mind to a calm state.

I'd frequently start a yoga session in a bad mood, without knowing exactly what was bothering me. Something just felt "off," and I had the urge to do something about it. Did you ever feel that way? It's a kind of nondescript, low grade angst that's hard to shake.

After yoga though, that feeling would disappear. I'd emerge into the very same world I came from, with all the same problems, except I no longer felt it was *urgent* to do anything. It's as if yoga gave my nervous system permission to chill out, breathe, and just think about things for a while.

I asked several instructors about this. They informed me that deep, yogic breathing takes you from a state of *doing* into a state of *being*. In other words, it turns off the false alarms that say you need to "do" something quickly to fix your life, and instead allows you to just be present in the moment. One of my instructors put it like this: "You go from *'Danger, Will Robinson!'* to *'Hey, relax, you've got everything you need right now.'*" (If you don't get the reference, it's from an old TV show called *Lost in Space* where the robot shouted *'Danger!'* while flailing his arms to warn Will about an urgent threat.)

The relevant point is that the right kind of breathing can take you from a state of *doing* to a state of *being*. Indulging your cravings is something people feel an "urgent" need to *do*, so making this transition lessens the urge. **I learned this breathing in yoga, but it's very easy to replicate on your own.** It seems it was the breathing which made all the difference, not the posing and stretching. I'll explain how shortly.

In sum, the overwhelming urge to indulge cravings appears to be, at least in part, a false activation of our emergency response system – a false alarm, if you will. The brain perceives something wrong and wants to *do* something to fix it and fix it fast. It then insists on consuming extra food to prepare. *"You're going to need more energy to deal with urgent threats, so you'd better ingest calories now! If you don't, you might starve or become too weak to deal with them."*

It's not rational, but that's the whole point. Indulging our cravings almost never is!

Turn off the nervous system's false alarms and the intensity of your cravings drops to a much more manageable level. That's why the friend I had lunch with no longer felt the desire to binge after yoga. She'd breathed her way through the "emergency."

Once I understood this, I recalled comments from dozens of clients who'd figured out how to accomplish the same thing in several different ways. It seems my friend wasn't alone in her discovery, and there was more than one way to calm your cravings.

Any method or practice that turns off the false alarms can work, but there are five methods which seem almost miraculous. In order of importance, they are:

a. Regular, reliable nutrition.

b. A simple breathing technique you can use at any time.

c. Inserting a few "decision-free" breaks during the day.

d. Falling in love with the journey *(a profound mindset shift away from weight loss and dieting.)*

e. Reframing stressful situations.

While regular, reliable nutrition is the most important and powerful, I'll cover it *last* because it's also the hardest to implement. The other four are perhaps 80% as effective, but because it's critical to find at least one that works for you, I'll start with the easiest ones. That said, please know if you've got erratic nutrition, or engage in extreme dieting, nothing I teach you will work. *If you want to defeat your cravings, it's essential to consume enough real food throughout the day.*

Now, at this point you might be thinking, *"Oh, c'mon, nobody in their right mind believes it's an emergency to get a donut!"* True that! But the point is, you don't have to *consciously* perceive the emergency and believe it's rational. Remember, these are *false* alarms. They're not about what you believe in your right mind, but what you *experience* in your warped one. You might not *think* there's an emergency behind your donut craving, but your reptilian brain may *feel* otherwise.

At minimum, please just accept that when people take the steps below, they find cravings easier to manage. After all, what if I'm right?

Here are the techniques in the order I suggest you try them.

BREATHING YOUR WAY THROUGH A CRAVING

How might you breathe if a hungry bear were chasing you?

As fast and as hard as you could!

You'd have to get as much oxygen into your lungs as quickly as humanly possible so you could feed your muscles and run like hell.

When you breathe fast and hard, your emergency system activates and presses for action to escape danger, fight off enemies, and gather scarce resources. Remember, food was scarce 100,000 years ago and your primitive brain still thinks it might be.

In contrast, when you're lying on the couch reading a book, you breathe much differently. Long, slow, relaxing breaths.

Breathing fast facilitates action, breathing slowly facilitates experiencing. Fast breaths validate false alarms, slower breaths turn them off! Another way to say this is that breathing fast makes you want to *do* stuff while breathing slowly helps you just *be*.

You can leverage this observation to calm down when you feel tempted, keep your wits about you, and turn off the urge to indulge. Breathe in slowly for a count of seven, then out even more slowly for a count of eleven. Repeat this three times. My friend Lori Hammond *(a hypnotist in Colorado)* first taught me this technique. She calls it a "seven-eleven breath" and it can be a miraculous part of the process.

Please take a moment to try it now.

I know it's more natural to continue reading but please do it anyway. It only takes 90 seconds.

You see, pausing when you have a very strong craving won't feel right at first either. It's much more natural to just eat when you have the urge. Pausing right now to try the seven-eleven breath begins to build your ability to pause at the moment of temptation when every bone in your body is screaming to indulge. You're going to need this mental muscle!

Most people are looking for a technique that feels natural and easy; one they really *want* to do. Unfortunately, we don't live in a natural food environment anymore, so you'll need to do something that feels unnatural *at first* if you want to master your cravings. So, practice this often until you get the hang of it.

Pausing will be uncomfortable at first. Just like writing down what your Pig says to get you to break the rules instead of eating when the craving hits. Do these things anyway. If you wait for an intervention that feels natural and easy, you're likely to be indulging your cravings forever.

I'll conclude with one last story about doing things to facilitate growth which might feel unnatural at first.

At 16 years old, I still hadn't gone out with a girl because I was painfully shy. Most other boys my age had been dating since junior high, but I'd never asked anyone out. Well, there was this girl named Karen who I really liked. My friend gave me her number. That night, I went downstairs to my father's office *(my power place)* to make the call. I must've been sitting on his couch staring at the phone for an hour, looking and feeling pathetic, when Dad walked in.

"What are you doing?" he asked.

"I really like this girl Karen and I want to ask her out," I replied.

"So why haven't you called her?"

"It doesn't feel right yet. I'm scared," I replied.

"Glenn, if you wait for it to *feel* right, you're going to be an old man before you get a date," he said.

So, I made the call.

It's a bit of a sad story because Karen rejected me, but I got over my fear of asking. That moment was the first time I understood some things are the right thing to do even if they don't feel right at first. It was a pivotal moment in the development of my life's philosophy. I learned that feelings aren't facts, so try to guide key decisions with your intellect, rather than allowing emotions to control you.

So, did you pause to try the seven-eleven breath?

I love you either way, but I really hope you did!

Next, we're going to add this breathing routine to the refutation process.

Previously when you heard your Pig Squealing to break your rules, you'd just write down what it said. But now I want you to take at least one seven-eleven breath before you write. Then write down the Squeal(s) and take at least one more seven-eleven breath before refuting them.

Adding seven-eleven breaths calms the sense of urgency and makes it easier to think straight during the refutation process. This results in a more powerful refutation as well as more immediate confidence in your ability to resist the craving.

Your breath is a very simple tool, and it's with you all the time. The trick is pausing long enough to use it to its fullest, especially when you don't want to!

BULK UP YOUR WILLPOWER WITH DECISION-FREE BREAK TIMES THROUGHOUT THE DAY

You will recall that willpower is like a full tank of gas you wake up with in the morning and burn throughout the day. There's a limit to how many good decisions you can make before you must sleep again to replenish.

I discussed this while persuading you that hard and fast rules eliminate decision making and preserve willpower for more important things. But did you know there are other very powerful implications of this understanding of willpower?

It turns out you can *restore* a good deal of your willpower by taking just a few decision-free breaks throughout the day. Even five minutes makes a difference.

See, every decision burns willpower, not just food decisions. For example, studies show that making people do math problems before offering them a marshmallow makes them significantly more likely to eat it.

You make many more decisions throughout the day than you realize, too.

Every time you get an email you decide whether to mark it as spam, respond to it, delegate it, defer it, act on it, or share it. Every time your children interrupt you to find out who's taking them to soccer practice, what they should wear, whether you can pick up their friend along the way, whether you'll stay and watch the game, etc., you're making decisions and burning willpower. Mary wants a team meeting at work? Well, what time can you coordinate that and who should you talk to first? Another set of decisions. Even using social media requires an endless series of decisions. Which posts and videos should you watch? Should you react to them? Which reaction do you choose – like, love, anger, cry, or care? What should you post?

We all live in a decision-making world. You're bombarded by decisions 24 x 7 x 365. Like it or not, each one eats up a little willpower.

But you can take a break! Put your phone in your desk drawer. Take a walk outside. Lay down and close your eyes for a few minutes. Heck, even going to the bathroom and sitting in the stall for five minutes without any devices helps more than you could imagine. *(A lot of busy mothers with young children use this trick to "steal" decision-free time.)*

Don't allow constant decision making to grind down your willpower day in and day out. Insert a few planned breaks into your day to restore and replenish. I tell most clients to start with five-minute decision-free breaks twice per day. No matter how busy you are, you can find this time. You'll probably make much better decisions throughout the rest of your day if you do, and that will save more time than it took to manufacture the breaks.

One quick aside about willpower before moving on: Because willpower is most plentiful in the morning, many people who struggle with nighttime overeating make significant progress by making their important food decisions before they start their day. Prepare your dinner and put it in containers first thing when you wake up. Make sure it's something you'll look forward to. Leave it someplace you'll see it when you get home, or at least leave a visible reminder that it's in the fridge, etc. This way you won't have to make a food decision when you walk in the door after a super-long day feeling depleted. And whenever you feel tempted out of the house, force yourself to think about what's waiting for you when you get home.

A few five-minute decision-free breaks each day can restore your willpower and determination. It really helps!

REFRAME STRESS TO OVERCOME CRAVINGS

It turns out the reptilian brain is capable of viewing virtually any situation as an emergency, especially if your Pig thinks it can use this as an excuse to get you to indulge. Luckily, you can use the refutations process to calm these kinds of false emergencies too.

The key, as with all Pig Squeals, is to recognize, articulate, and refute what the Pig is saying, particularly its conclusion that the stress is a reason to break the rules. In the process you'll likely calm yourself regarding the stressor itself, but that's not the goal. Rather, you must first and foremost invalidate the Pig's argument that the presence of stress is a reason to indulge. You need to sever the link between stress and overeating.

For example, perhaps you're way behind on paying your mortgage, just got a notice of foreclosure, and find yourself on the verge of bankruptcy. Your Pig will undoubtedly say the *only* way to feel better is to stuff yourself with Pig Slop. *"There's SO much financial stress in your life right now, and literally nothing feels good. It's unbearable. The only possible pleasure you can get right now is from eating Pig Slop! Let's go get some. You deserve a break from the torture, don't you?"*

How can you stop the Pig in its tracks?

Refuting the idea that Pig Slop is the *only* possible pleasure would sever the link.

Refuting the idea that Pig Slop is a reward and not a punishment would sever the link.

Refuting the idea that you "deserve" Pig Slop by explaining what you *really* deserve would sever the link.

None of these things would remove the pending bankruptcy, but they'd prevent you from having an overeating episode and help you stay on plan, which, in turn, would help you stay present and able to use your problem-solving abilities. And remember, if you have six problems and then you overeat, you'll have seven problems when you're done.

Once the link is severed, you'll naturally feel calmer because you'll be safe from the Pig. However, you can proceed to refute the ideas which are aggravating the stress. Is it really unbearable? Why or why not. What are you imagining is going to happen versus what really could, and probably would happen? Refute, refute, refute.

Speaking of life stressors, there was a time in my life when I was $700,000+ in debt, behind on my payables by nine months, with virtually no income coming and thinking, *"Some guys in white suits with mustaches are going to come to take away my furniture, computers, car, and kick me out of my house."* It never happened. If you're going through serious financial struggles, you might want to listen to this teleconference I did in 2009. It was about recovering from the $700,000 debt. Thousands of people attended and, for many years later, I received detailed thank-you notes from people all over the world. It might help you with any related false activation of your emergency system. A recording of this teleconference is available in the free reader bonuses on the website. (www.DefeatYourCravings.com)

This works for virtually any type of stress, but let's go through a few very specific and common examples.

Managing Financial Stress Before It Kills You

The Pig says, "*There's SO much financial stress in our lives right now, and literally nothing feels good. It's unbearable. The only possible pleasure available to you now is to eat Pig Slop! Let's go get some right now. You deserve a break from the torture, don't you?*"

Well, first, would Pig Slop really make you feel better?

Things might be bad, but overeating isn't a treat; it's a punishment that will only make things worse. If you abstain from Slop, you might still go broke, but if you indulge the craving, you could become fat, sick, *and* broke. That certainly wouldn't feel better. I know — been there, done that, got the T-shirt *(way back in 2002)*!

Also, the high you'll get from consuming sugar and white flour is short-lived. A recent meta-analysis of 31 studies and 1,259 participants concluded that people are not only significantly more fatigued and less alert an hour after intake of refined carbohydrates, but it was also questionable whether the carb intake improved their mood for even a short period (Mantantzis et al. 2019).

Your dopamine system also becomes somewhat depleted during this crash, making your ability to think positively almost non-existent. Conclusion? Pig Slop doesn't make you feel better!

Second, is Pig Slop really the only pleasure available to you during a financial crisis? I think not. As far as I know there are still hundreds of free parks around the country where you can get outside, breathe, and relax in nature. There are also plenty of dogs to pet and smile at on the streets, libraries where you can read books for free, people to hug, children who won't charge you to play with them, naps you don't have to pay for, friends who might welcome a phone call, etc., etc., etc. Not to mention all the healthy, delicious on-plan food you can eat! No, Pig Slop is far from the only pleasure available when you're broke!

Lastly, when you're suffering financial stress, the Pig says you deserve some Slop, but what do you *really* deserve? I might suggest it's freedom from bloating, digestive distress, constantly worrying about your health and your weight, how to make up for the indulgence, how to hide the evidence, as well as freedom from obsessing about exactly how much Slop you can get away with before you put the Pig back in its cage. Peace of mind – that's what you deserve!

See how this works?

You begin with the Pig's best shot to get you to indulge because of stress, and methodically disempower its logic, just like with any other refutation.

How to "Cope" with Any Emotion WIthout Overeating

Let's say the love of your life threatens to leave you. Your Pig will say nobody can be expected to bear this without Slop. After all, what cold and cruel person would deny you that, given what you're going through? It says you must go out and get some Slop today, tomorrow, and every day until your relationship is secure once again.

Well, facing the loss of the love of your life might be your worst nightmare, but do you know what's even worse than that? Facing this threat *and* threats to your health, fitness, and ability to concentrate on communicating and problem solving your way through it. In fact, I'd say your best chance of keeping love rests with eating healthier than you ever have before. I don't know about you, but even if the love of my life did leave me, I wouldn't want to go through the next few months in a food coma. I'd want my wits about me to fix things.

Do you see how this is done?

Whatever seems so awful, figure out how your Pig is trying to turn it into an opportunity to indulge in a whole pile of Slop. Then refute that argument. You might not solve the problem, but you'll sever the link that turns emotional problems into big hairy overeating episodes. Capiche?

Okay, next we'll turn to the most-effective-but-hardest-to-implement way to make your emergency response system set off a lot fewer false alarms!

The End of Yo-Yo Dieting

"When she was good, she was very good indeed, but when she was bad, she was horrid!"

Henry Wadsworth Longfellow

In the poem "There Was a Little Girl," Henry Wadsworth Longfellow unwittingly captured the classic overeater's relationship with food. Now, if you're like most people who struggle with overeating, you're probably a great dieter too. I'm guessing you're capable of being very strict for a while to "make up for" equally intense periods of overeating. You probably cling to memories of successful dieting as the thing that's going to "save" you. No matter how badly you eat, no matter how much weight you gain, no matter how far down the give-in-to-the-cravings hole you may sink, you probably believe you'll be able to fix things quickly with your dieting skills. If so, welcome to the club!

At first, this mentality seems perfectly reasonable to most people. After all, their histories are littered with a roller coaster of ups and downs, and *in the early stages*, they recall repeatedly dieting themselves back down to their desired weight. The Pig is quick to cite this as proof the diet-binge cycle works and says there's nothing to worry about because you can always repair the damage later.

In the beginning, it's usually just five or ten pounds of weight gain. But as time progresses, the cravings get worse, you indulge more intensely, losing weight gets harder, and you have a lot more to lose. Before you know it, it's 20, then 40, and then *(for some)* 100 pounds or more. Nobody starts out thinking, *"I'd like to gain a hundred pounds and lose it again, that will be fun,"* but you become immersed in this feast-or-famine cycle, and your brain begins to experience that food may be an *urgent* matter. This makes the cravings a lot harder to resist.

With time, normal metabolic aging also takes hold, and advances in the Big Food industry make hyper-palatable food-like substances even harder to resist – *the chips you binge on today are more addictive than those you ate 20 years ago.*

Yo-yoing up and down also slows the metabolism, making the "super-diet" strategy progressively less feasible. The longer this cycle goes on, the more trapped you feel, until, eventually, you find yourself thinking about food almost all the time, crowding out your more valuable, life-enhancing thoughts.

The only way out is to step off the feast-or-famine roller coaster and swear off dieting for good, but most people fight this tooth and nail.

This is a very difficult chapter for me to write because, first and foremost, I must respect your autonomy when it comes to food. Your rules and dietary philosophy must be your decision entirely, because if it's not, your Pig will convince you to reject "Glenn's diet." Then you'll be back where you started. Autonomy in your food choice is pivotal.

Yet, at the same time, I'd be remiss if I didn't tell you that across almost 2,000 clients, my team and I have seen approximately *double* the success rate for people who don't skip meals and regularly nourish their bodies. From my experience, a greater number of people genuinely defeat their cravings in the long-term by embracing a very reasonable diet with slow and steady weight loss.

What does that mean in practical terms?

Unless a doctor advises you otherwise, it usually means three or more meals per day, spread throughout a no-less-than-12-hour eating window. It also means losing no more than a pound or two per week, and adjusting your food intake upward if weight starts to come off too quickly. (*People with 70+ pounds to lose sometimes can proceed at a faster pace the first few months.*) Finally, it means avoiding extreme diets which may be deficient in vital macronutrients and micronutrients.

What about intermittent fasting?

Intermittent fasting works best with the *Defeat Your Cravings* method if you first wait until you've largely defeated your cravings for a span of approximately six months. Many clients, however, insist on implementing an intermittent fasting protocol right away anyway. These individuals prefer to restrict their eating to a very small window, often allowing themselves just one meal per day. My team and I sometimes jokingly call this "binging on a schedule" but most clients don't think this is funny because they're very attached to the intermittent fasting idea. My team and I say it anyway because we want to force people to, at a minimum, think carefully about their choices in this area.

Melanie Avalon, the host of the *Intermittent Fasting Podcast*, was once my guest on an extremely well-attended webinar about this controversial topic. During the event she agreed it was better for people to ease into intermittent fasting if they'd been eating a lot of processed foods up until that point, especially foods containing sugar and flour. She said it can take quite some time to get these things out of the system and become "fat adapted," which she says is required to settle into intermittent fasting successfully.

So, if intermittent fasting is your thing, great! But I suggest you wait six months before implementing it so you can successfully adopt the *Defeat Your Cravings* method first. You may still succeed if you do decide to try intermittent fasting right away, it's just a higher mountain to climb.

Full fasting that lasts 24 hours or longer, regardless of the variety (*juice, water, etc.*), just doesn't seem to work. It helps with cravings in the short run, and might have medical benefits, but from what I've observed with overeaters it makes cravings a lot worse down the road. I might venture to say I've never seen someone succeed in defeating their cravings if they engage in full fasts right out of the gate. For this reason, I recommend getting your cravings under control for nine months before trying to reintroduce full fasting into your routine.

Regardless of when and how you choose to eat, making sure you get regular, reliable nutrition is a critical part of the solution. So, too, is checking to ensure you're not deficient in any key nutrients. I'm happiest when people consult with a licensed, experienced dietitian with relevant expertise on this front because I've found most people *think* they're eating healthy, but an expert will inevitably point out key dietary mistakes. If you'd prefer not to go this route, there are several online nutritional calculators you can use to check the nutritional and caloric value of the food you're consuming.

Regularly fortifying your body with the right nutrition, aiming for slow, steady weight loss, and swearing off dieting for good – all help make food a much less urgent matter. This calms the reptilian brain, weakens cravings, and makes the whole process of defeating your food cravings a lot easier.

How To Fall In Love With The Weight Loss Journey

You can and should take things a step further if you're willing. You can fall in love with the weight loss journey itself!

What does that mean?

There are at least a dozen incredible benefits that come from mastering your cravings which have nothing to do with weight loss. You can consciously and purposefully cultivate appreciation for these benefits.

For example, most people begin to feel they really can be the master of their own destiny when they can stick to even one food rule. As the adage goes, you are what you eat. In fact, feeding ourselves is a primal force for self-esteem, and when we can successfully implement one food rule, this sense of empowerment can begin to positively impact the rest of your life. Such an accomplishment can inspire hope, enthusiasm, and confidence, not only with food but in your ability to achieve your personal, professional, and social goals. It's not uncommon for people to report all sorts of improvements in their lives, even after just a few weeks.

It feels much, *much* better to be the master of your own food choices than a slave to your impulses!

Beyond this, following a well-thought-out set of rules begins to free people from their food obsession, leaving them with time to enjoy their family, friends, work, and leisure activities. It also tends to eliminate the need to lie about and/ or hide what you're eating, which creates a sense of pride and joy rather than embarrassment and shame.

Eating better also often improves important biomarkers and health risks. Depending on the specific changes you make, indicators such as blood pressure, diabetes markers, inflammation, joint pain, cardiovascular risk factors, can all reach normal, healthy levels. Often people can reduce and/ or eliminate medications and unwanted side effects – *always with a doctor's supervision* – way before all the weight is off.

Factors such as increased energy, ease of breathing, radiant skin tone, and positive thinking can also improve dramatically. And even though body image is the last thing to shift, most people can't help but smile when their clothes start to fit better, and others start to notice less bloating in their faces. You don't have to be at goal weight to experience improvements in these areas.

Cultivating a heightened awareness of all this is the best retort when your Pig Squeals, *"This isn't fast enough, you've got to restrict to get the weight off quickly!"* Disallowing panic about weight loss reduces the false sense of emergency that feeds the overeating cycle.

Paradoxically, the back door to weight loss is to take the focus off weight loss. A weight loss focus makes food and eating too much an urgent matter. Panicking about the scale generally makes it go up, not down! Fall in love with the weight loss journey instead of weight loss.

"But, Glenn, you don't understand, I have a wedding (or another event) to attend, and I look hideous. I can't be seen like this, it would be too humiliating, so I have no choice but to lose weight fast!"

First, many if not most of the clients I've seen who have attempted to lose weight quickly for an upcoming event often wind up attending the event heavier than their starting weight, or gaining even more weight once the event is over. Statistically, it's a losing strategy.

If your Pig is still squealing about this, please take a deep breath and conjure the image of someone you know and respect who has approximately the same amount of weight to lose as you do. If you don't know anyone personally, a celebrity, other public figure, or even a fictional character will do. Once you have the person in mind, ask yourself if you'd tell this person not to go to a wedding because they were too fat? Would you say they should be embarrassed to show their face? Would you shun them, and refuse to hug or kiss them hello until they lost enough weight? Would you call them ugly and disgusting?

I think not!

In contrast, you'd probably be really supportive if you knew they'd settled into a slow, steady, reliable, and calm journey toward weight loss and, more importantly, permanent health. You'd hug, love, and encourage them. You'd help them feel proud of their choices. You'd be a loving friend, colleague, etc.

Now, how about doing that for yourself?

I've yet to hear anyone I've walked through this exercise return to say the event was humiliating or embarrassing. I've only been thanked for the encouragement.

The takeaway is that panicking about weight loss only digs you deeper into the overeating cycle. Find a way to make defeating your cravings your primary goal. I know it's hard, and a very different way of living your life, but the rewards are incredible. Plus, the alternative approach hasn't ever fully worked for you, or you wouldn't be reading this book! Right?

The Pig says it's not possible to shift your mindset, but what if it were possible?

ELIMINATING OTHER PROBLEMS THAT SET OFF FALSE EMERGENCY REACTIONS

There are six additional things you can do to minimize false emergency reactions in your reptilian brain. I didn't include them in the "fabulous four" above because they're a little more difficult to work on and not always entirely in your control. Nevertheless, you should know that getting enough sleep, exercise, and human contact will calm your nervous system and make it less likely to set off a false alarm. So, too, will meditation, yoga, and time outside, which are all shown to increase natural dopamine response *(a neurotransmitter responsible for feeling pleasure and an overall sense of satisfaction)*.

I recommend you focus on as much of the "fabulous four" *(breathing, decision-free breaks, reframing stressful situations, and falling in love with the journey)* with the goal of becoming exceptionally good with at least one of them. Just keep the rest in mind and do what you can, when you can, to improve. There are literally hundreds of books you can read on meditation, yoga, enjoying nature, building your social support network, etc., so I'm not going to focus on these areas in this book.

Now, let's move on to amping up your motivation.

To download a free cheat sheet on the process of turning off false alarms please visit www.DefeatYourCravings.com.

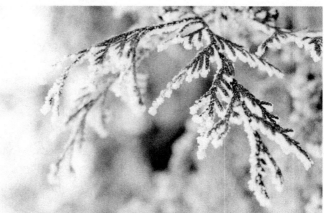

CULTIVATE POWERFUL MOTIVATION

BEFORE YOU BEGIN

> Before you begin working on improving your motivation, it's important for you to feel that your food rules are exceptionally doable – especially when you don't feel like complying!

Amping up motivation can be very helpful, and it certainly makes the process of defeating your cravings feel a lot better. I'll therefore present a detailed and unique motivational technique below. But unfortunately, no matter what you do, motivation waxes and wanes like the tides – *nobody can stay motivated 100% of the time*. When it's high, it's much easier for most people to stay on plan. The trick is adopting a plan you can stick to even when you *don't* feel like it!

One reason I want you to begin with one simple rule is because it's a relatively low bar you can consistently achieve no matter how motivated you feel. When the Pig says, *"Screw it, just do it, who cares?"* you must be able to say, *"I don't need to care because it's pretty easy to comply!"* For this reason, setting the bar at a reasonable level makes you much more likely to consistently stay on-plan over time. This is key, because observing yourself doing something consistently will help change your identity. The rules become a sacred part of you. They also become second nature – something you just *do* without having to think about all the time. Then you can start to raise the bar slowly over time.

On the other hand, if you start this with a high initial bar, there'll come a day when you just can't find your mojo, and you'll have a much harder time saying *"No!"* to the Pig when it Squeals. Breaking your food rules is a very bad idea because, as you'll learn in a later chapter on the science of habit extinction, you'll reset the extinction curve to day zero each time, dooming you to a longer, harder struggle against your cravings. This is how people get trapped in a downward food cravings spiral.

> **Hitting a low bar with consistency is much better than hitting a high bar sporadically.**

Consistency creates lasting change.

Therefore, please review your rules one last time and ask yourself if they're strong enough to make a difference, but still easy enough to comply with when it's the last thing on earth you feel like doing. Then adjust accordingly.

As a quick aside, you can and should refute the Pig when motivation is low, too; just expect it to be a bit more work to achieve. For example, if you're feeling like death warmed over and the Pig says you just don't feel like staying on plan, say, *"Why do I have to feel like it? I make intellectual decisions about my most important food choices, not emotional ones!"*

Once you're confident you'll be able to execute your food rules even in a foul mood, it's safe to move on.

Note

I was first exposed to the idea of a low bar in B.J. Fogg's book **Tiny Habits.**

WHY YOU NEED POWERFUL MOTIVATION

It's one thing to know what to do, but quite another to get yourself to do it. For this reason, it's important to ask *why* you want to defeat your cravings? I know it seems silly, but in the absence of powerfully articulated reasons, all the disciplines I've described so far are like installing a squadron of food police in your head. It might scare you straight for a while, but without powerful reasons pulling you forward, you won't want to keep running from the food police forever.

Furthermore, the research we did with almost 800 clients, readers, and prospects suggests simple motivational answers like "I'd like to lose some weight" or "I'd like to look better in clothes" are great for getting started but insufficient for permanent change. The closer you get to your goal, the more these motivations fade. For example, when you hit your goal weight, the motivation to lose weight disappears entirely, and the halo effect of people noticing you're getting thinner will have long since passed, so you won't have much to help you stay thin. So, what kind of motivation is more likely to work longer-term?

MOTIVATION THAT DOESN'T SUCK: HOW TO FIND SUSTAINABLE MOTIVATION FOR YOUR PERSONAL NEEDS

Our research suggested that there were three essential types of motivation found primarily in people who've reached their goal and kept it off for approximately one year or more:

01. the desire to be free from food obsession,

02. the need to put an end to yo-yo dieting once and for all, and

03. the fear of being diagnosed with serious health conditions.

Essential Motivations

The first and strongest of these was the desire to permanently end food obsession. People who were able to stay at their goal weight felt that their food thoughts had taken over too much of their lives, crowding out the ability to be present for more important things. They'd often reached their goal as a by-product of this motivation, not by focusing on weight loss itself. In short, they wanted continued mental freedom above all else.

Coming in at an extremely close second was the desire to be done with dieting forever. Many said they'd already tried virtually every diet available, that being on a diet "sucked," and they were beyond exhausted from having to starve themselves at regular intervals.

Finally, the third motivation which helped people to achieve their goal and stay there was the fear of an existing health condition, the likelihood of developing a potentially serious illness or disease. Many had close relatives they'd seen suffer the ravages of diabetes, disability from strokes and heart attacks, kidney problems, and worse. Often their doctor had already given them a warning that they were going down the same road. Awareness of the risks alone wasn't enough, however. These outcomes needed to seem like exquisitely real possibilities from personal experience.

To recapitulate, my most successful readers and clients all seem to have achieved their success NOT via a focus on weight loss itself but based on the desire for freedom from food obsession and yo-yo dieting, as well as fear of serious health conditions which had impacted them (or a loved one) personally.

Also, please note that not everyone who succeeded had adopted one of these essential motivations at the outset. There were a wide variety of incentives – *mostly the desire to lose weight and look better* – that got people started. But as they obtained a degree of success, these initial motivations gave way to one or more of the essential three above.

Nice-to-Have Motivations

Lastly, there were six types of motivation that I categorize as "nice-to-haves" that helped people stick to their plan. These included:

a. Having more energy

b. Becoming a healthy role model for children and family

c. Alleviating or eliminating the possibility of a minor health condition (*joint pain, arthritis, skin problems, etc.*)

d. Looking good in clothing and to enjoy shopping

e. Finding meaning in previous suffering by telling one's story publicly

f. Eliminating the hypocrisy gap (*for health professionals, personal trainers, nutritionists, etc., e.g., "Nobody hires a fat personal trainer."*)

Having one or more of these "nice to have" motivations can substitute for the essentials as you begin, but it's necessary to also adopt at least one of the essential motivations as you get some success behind you.

Motivation That Sucks

Finally, there was one type of motivation that was more predictive of failure than success – *shame!* Shame gets people to "start their diet" but, from all the evidence I've seen, is simply not sustainable. Most people operating from a sense of shame seem to quit before making much progress. This phenomenon is seen across all genders and ages but is a particularly common among younger women. Everything we do in the *Defeat Your Cravings* method is therefore intended to minimize this pernicious emotion.

MOST MOTIVATION ADVICE LACKS THIS CRITICAL COMPONENT

Most motivational advice in the healthy eating space consists largely of asking the question, *"Why do you want to be thin and fit?"* You're asked to consider your "Big Why" without specific prompts to link to the *entirety* of your life. This doesn't make sense because healthy eating impacts a *lot* more than just weight. Moreover, what you really need is *specific* motivation to engage in a specific set of behaviors – *to comply with your specific food rules* – not just general motivation to eat well. Finally, as reviewed above, most motivational work doesn't account for the fact that certain types of motivation are enough to get you started on your plan but fade quickly as you approach your goal.

The *Defeat Your Cravings* motivation method is food rule specific. You'll begin with the all-important question: **"What might life be like in one year if you complied 100% with your specific food rule or set of rules?"** This question draws motivation from your underlying beliefs – *both conscious and unconscious* – about what your *specific* food rules will *specifically* do for you. This is a crucial framework.

You see, every decision in life defines a unique path by influencing future decisions, so following even one rule can make a giant difference in one year. Let's consider this rule: *"I'll never go back for seconds again."* You might think this wouldn't impact weight loss and health too much because it only limits the volume of food you consume since you can still eat whatever you want. However, limits on food volume shouldn't be dismissed lightly. Many people consume two or three times as much as they need, or more! *So even one simple rule like, "I'll never again go back for seconds," can have a profound impact on an individual's future.*

Plus, when people don't follow *any* rules for a long time, they start to feel out of control and helpless, like some external force has taken over their eating. The

Pig then gains prominence: *"Who cares, just eat whatever you want, and as much as you want!"* Things can easily spiral downward from there.

However, the moment you can prove that just one simple rule works for you, a newfound sense of confidence begins to replace those awful feelings of inadequacy, eventually turning into a positive snowball effect. You find yourself more present, with more energy, and feeling less bloated. You think, *"This is great! I could do more!"* So, you draft *another* rule: *"I'll always start my days with a 16-ounce green smoothie."* This, too, then becomes a positive snowball, and you begin to address even more cravings.

A year later you've not only lost weight, but perhaps your knees no longer hurt, and your skin has cleared up. Maybe you've become intimate with your spouse again. Perhaps your digestion is a billion times better. You spontaneously get down on the floor to play with your kids *(or grandkids)*, go for walks, hikes, play sports, are more present, etc. You sleep better and may even become more productive at work, which can impact your career and finances.

The point is, complying with even one rule produces a series of positive impacts across your whole life which you must capture in your "Big Why." The Big Why is your imagination about what your rule-compliant life will be like in the future. The Pig will scream "This is impossible! There's no way you'll ever make it that long, so it's not even worth doing the exercise." But what if you *did* make it that long despite the Pig's protests? What might change for the better?

Sometimes people can't get past the idea that they'll never be able to defeat their cravings for an entire year. If that's you, scale back to something you believe is possible. Start with a month, or a week, or even just 72 hours. It's critical you believe in your "Big Why," so turning it into a "Little Why" until you get some momentum is perfectly fine. I've even seen people succeed with as little as a ten-hour timeframe, focusing mostly on the physical changes they'll experience in their digestion and mood once the most recent round of Pig Slop passes through them. Then they created a "Bigger Why" afterward.

DISCOVER A "BIGGER WHY" THAN YOU'VE EVER HAD BEFORE!

It's important to note these motivational exercises are a lot better *demonstrated* than described. For this reason, I've recorded several full-length motivational interviews where you can listen to me guiding people through the process firsthand. You can listen for free when you join the reader bonus list at www.DefeatYourCravings.com

The first almost magical motivation question to ask yourself is: **"What might my life be like in one year if I comply 100% with my rules?"** However, let's not stop there. Instead, prompt yourself to imagine what things will be like *in very specific areas* that span the entirety of your life.

Imagine it's one full year from now, and you've succeeded despite your Pig's best efforts. You've complied with your rule(s) 100% of the time for one entire year and doing so has led to a positive series of changes that radically improved your life.

For each life area below, try to imagine the best possible, yet still believable, result. Imagine failure is no longer an option and success has already been achieved. Your Pig will say this is impossible, but what if the exact opposite were true – what if you could not only do it, but what if it were actually impossible for you to break your rules!? You should assume that you'll see a dramatic difference in at least some areas after a full year of success. Also, try to use specific words that excite and motivate you. So, for example, it's not, *"I feel more confident,"* but rather, *"My confidence is soaring! There's no stopping me!"*

How Will Your Confidence Skyrocket?

As compared to how you're feeling today, how confident would you look and feel in the mirror after one full year of success? How, specifically, does this manifest? Do you hold yourself differently, stand more upright, or enter a room with more confidence? Perhaps your eyes look clearer or you're smiling more. Maybe it's just in how you choose to dress. What's the difference?

Everything Should Improve for You Physically

As compared to today, what changes in your physical body do you see in the mirror after one full year of success? Perhaps your digestion is better, or your skin is clearer. Maybe you envision feeling less physical pain, agitation, or inflammation. Do your joints ache less, or not at all? Perhaps your face looks less bloated. What's the difference? Look carefully within your imagination and take notes on the details. Use exciting words and specifics. Don't just say, *"I look good,"* say, *"I look absolutely amazing! I can't believe it's me! I'm so gorgeous and proud!"*

Become Free from Constant food Thoughts

As compared to today, what changes in mental freedom do you imagine feeling after one full year of success? What might it feel like to be completely free from food obsession? Use exciting words. It's not, *"I am free of the mental obsession,"* but rather, *"My mind is clear, focused, present, and purposeful. I can concentrate my mental energy on important things like my children, my job, and my friends. I can't believe it!"*

Dramatically Reduce Health Concerns

As compared to today, what changes in your health concerns might you imagine have begun to develop after one year of success? Are these concerns completely gone? What's it like to have so much less anxiety about this? Use exciting words and specifics. What's the best possible, yet still believable, result? For example, *"I can't even imagine having a heart attack now because I feel so healthy, fit, and strong!"*

Seriously Boost Your Energy Levels

As compared to today, what changes in energy levels do you imagine might begin to develop after one full year of success? Most people find themselves with a *lot* more physical energy at this point. Use exciting words. Don't just say,

"I have more energy," say, *"I have boundless energy and have become a real dynamo, doing things I only dreamed of before like _____, _____, and _____."* Describe exactly what you'd be doing with all the added energy!

Enjoy Stronger Relationships

As compared to today, what changes in your relationships do you imagine might develop after one full year of success? How might things be different with colleagues, friends, peers, children, spouse, and family? This extends to your social life, too. In your imagination, look carefully and note the difference. Use specific names that will act as a reminder later. And of course, use big and exciting words. Don't just say, *"I'm closer with my spouse,"* say, *"I can't believe it, but we've been intimate again and I love it!"*

Look Good in Anything You Wear

As compared to today, what clothing choice changes do you imagine you've begun to make after one full year of success? Many people find themselves choosing more attractive clothes and enjoying more options because of the changes they envision in their body and confidence levels. In your imagination, look carefully and take notes. Which clothes do you already have hanging in your closet which you *would* wear if you felt more confident about your shape? What clothing choices might you make if you dropped a dress size? Two sizes? Use big, exciting words! Don't just say, *"I'd wear that pair of jeans in the closet."* Instead say, *"I'd wear that sexy pair of black jeans with the hole in the knee that constantly turns heads!"*

Make More Money and Accomplish More in Your Career

As compared to today, what changes in career and personal finances might you imagine would start to develop after one full year of success? Some people imagine they'd be more likely to act on financial and/or career projects because of their additional energy and confidence. In your imagination, look carefully and note the difference. If you do see a difference in your financial and/or career activities, try to quantify how much of a financial impact there might be. Be specific. Imagine some things you could do to improve your career and/or finances if you felt like you ruled the world – a feeling which often comes when you learn to control your Pig! Use big, exciting words! Don't say, *"I will make $10,000 more per year,"* say, *"The $10,000 extra I'll make every year has taken the edge off of my/our financial situation. I feel calm about money for the first time in my life, and it's only going to get better. After ten years I will have earned $100,000 that I wouldn't have if I had kept overeating – it's amazing!"*

Enjoy Exercise, Sports, the Great Outdoors, and Other Physical Activities

As compared to today, what changes in your exercise, sports participation, and/or physical activity level do you imagine might begin to develop after one full year of success? Some people don't wish to incorporate this into their lives, but if you do, think carefully about what might happen, talk about why it's important, and note the difference. Maybe you'd add a short workout session each day. Or participating in a sport you've always wanted to do. Remember, in one year you'll probably be in a completely different place with your confidence and physical well-being, so give yourself permission to dream. Use big, exciting words! Don't say, *"I'll go back to hiking with the kids again,"* say, *"I will hike Soldier's Dome with the kids on July 12th next year to celebrate. I can see myself and the kids with their arms high in the air to celebrate our victorious ascent!"*

PUTTING IT ALL TOGETHER

Look at your notes on all the above and try to incorporate it into one statement, perhaps one-half to one full page long. **Make sure you're stating everything in the positive, and in the present tense as if it has already happened.** It's not, "I want to stop passing mounds of food through my body and feeling so gross and disgusting," but rather, *"I naturally eat normal volumes of food and feel free of digestive distress."* It's not, "I wish I weren't such a fat, lazy, blob," but rather, *"I enjoy exercising and do so consistently."*

My own "Big Why" statement follows, but please remember, this is just for illustration purposes! Your "Big Why" may be entirely different and should be drawn from answers to *your* rules-specific questions above.

GLENN'S EXAMPLE: *"I comply with my food plan and refute the Pig 100% of the time so I can walk in the world as a healthy, confident, thin man, who radiates a smiling presence. I'm free from worry about heart attacks, strokes, diabetes, dementia, and cancer. I'm confident in my ability to have a romantic and passionate relationship with a woman I love. I'll maintain my ideal weight forever. I'm leading my company to true greatness as someone who walks the walk and doesn't have to look over his shoulder while he eats. I inspire millions and am a productivity machine with a secure and substantial salary. I never have to recover from a meal, always have the energy to get things done, and track my exercise for steady progress! I religiously do my physical therapy and inversion table work, so I'm completely free of sciatic numbness. My body feels like it did when I was in my early twenties! This is why I comply with my food plan and refute the Pig 100% of the time."*

Please note I've added a "commitment statement" to the beginning and end of my "Big Why." This helps stamp in the connection between the future I'm looking to achieve, complying with my food plan, and refuting the Pig at every turn.

THE BIG "WHY NOT"

When we did our first set of follow-ups to check on the results of my previous coaching program, I'd thought the number one predictor of success would be how seriously people had taken the Big Why exercise. I was wrong! The Big Why did indeed predict success, but an even stronger predictor was what I call the "Big Why Not" – a detailed vision of what might happen five, ten, or even 15 years down the road if the Pig is *not* caged, kind of like the "ghost of Christmas future" in Charles Dickens' famous novella *A Christmas Carol*.

It turns out most people tend to think it's okay to put off improving their eating because they figure they can just hold the status quo for "a little while longer." But the truth for most is that if they're not getting better, they're getting worse, and deep down they know it.

"Things alter for the worse spontaneously, if they be not altered for the better designedly."

Francis Bacon

So, if you're feeling brave enough to face the ghost of Christmas future, then go through the same exact questions above, except change "after one full year of success" to "after *ten* years of letting the Pig do whatever it wants to." To spare you the need to page backward through the prompts above:

- ☑ What would happen to you physically?
- ☑ To your confidence?
- ☑ Your sense of mental freedom?
- ☑ Your energy levels?
- ☑ Relationships?
- ☑ Clothing?
- ☑ Career and finances?
- ☑ Exercise, sports participation, and physical well-being?

Feel free to skip this exercise if it sounds too painful. But if you choose to do it, be specific and detailed enough so you can really "scare yourself straight."

Then, when you're done, ask yourself what might be the opposite of each painful thing you envisioned? It will always be a positive element you might want to strive for. Does it make sense to incorporate this into your "Big Why?" If so, then add the "Big Why Not" to your "Big Why!"

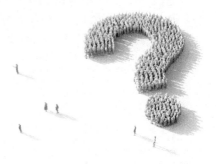

PUT AN END TO SHAME

In our extensive research, *shame* is a very ineffective motivation. It might get you started, but virtually nobody who has permanently managed their cravings has used shame to get to their goal weight and maintain it. It seems *shame* spirals in on itself when you focus on it, and this is almost inevitably self-destructive in the long run.

Yet, if you look at any formerly obese person's face you can almost always see residues of shame. It can be very pernicious and persistent. So how do you rid yourself of it?

First, make a list of *all* successes you've had with your eating, regardless of how long they lasted, and regardless of how tiny they may have been. For example: *"I stopped overeating on weekdays for a few months last year,"* or *"I don't eat my kid's leftovers anymore,"* or *"I only eat sugar on holidays and immediate family birthdays."*

Then, for each success, ask yourself whether you initially thought you'd be able to accomplish it. For example: *"I never thought I could get through a full week at work without indulging,"* or *"I was really convinced I was hopelessly addicted to sugar but proved myself wrong. I did it for a few days, so it's obviously not hopeless."*

Then, think about any successes *unrelated* to weight loss or eating you've had in the past. Say how each of them surprised you too.

Third, articulate the Squeals which perpetuate shame. For example, *"You've made a million promises to yourself and broken them, so you're obviously incapable of eating well for any length of time. It's just pathetic that you're even trying. You're hopeless."*

Then – *you know what I'm going to say* – refute these Squeals! I discussed the refutation for this particular Squeal previously, but it's also in the Appendix if you need it.

Finally, if you haven't done the "Falling in Love with the Weight Loss Journey" exercise, then do so now.

Earlier I suggested that you should first think of somebody you respect who's about your weight and size. You can use a celebrity or even a fictional character if need be. Would you tell this person not to go to a wedding because they were too heavy? Tell them they shouldn't dare show their face? Would you shun them until they lost enough weight? Would you call them ugly and disgusting? No! You'd be loving and supportive, helping them to act constructively and move toward their goal. Now, how about doing that for yourself?

It seems like a trite exercise, but if you're feeling ashamed of your eating, weight, or body, it's really very powerful.

Okay, now that you've been through the motivational exercises, it's time to review your "Big Why" one last time, then make concrete, practical plans to program it into your life!

REVIEWING FOR ESSENTIAL MOTIVATION

Remember, the most successful cravings defeaters all seem to have achieved their success NOT via a focus on weight loss per se, but rather based on the desire for freedom from food obsession and torturous yo-yo dieting, as well as avoiding serious health complications.

"Nice-to-have" helper motivations included having more energy; being a role model for children and family; alleviating less serious health conditions like joint pain, arthritis, or skin problems; looking good in clothing and enjoying shopping again; telling one's story to inspire others; and, for health professionals, personal trainers, etc., eliminating the hypocrisy gap.

Lastly, shame clearly needs to be eliminated to whatever extent possible.

So, before going forward, do you have at least one essential motivation represented in your "Big Why?" What about the nice-to-have motivations? Having one or more "nice-to-haves" can substitute for an essential motivation as you begin, provided you keep in mind it will be necessary to shift as you get some success behind you. And have you eliminated shame from your "Big Why" statement?

Finally, read through your "Big Why" one more time to see if you genuinely believe complying with your food plan will get you there in one full year. Adjust as necessary.

PROGRAMMING YOUR BIG WHY INTO YOUR LIFE

Doing your motivational exercises and writing your Big Why statement for the first time should be a very pleasant and motivating experience. You'll probably feel happier than you've felt in a long time. However, the Big Why functions more like a vitamin than an antibiotic. It works its magic by repeated exposure, day in and day out, rather than in one short course of "treatment."

"It takes constant repetition to force alien concepts on reluctant minds," said Freud, who I am *not* a fan of, but who nonetheless captured a fundamental truth in this statement. It's important that you repeatedly expose yourself to the "Big Why" over the long haul, especially the first few months you're working on defeating your cravings.

There are several ways to do this.

Since you'll be reading your food plan out loud each morning for the first few months, you can just add the Big Why to this routine. Read it slowly, emotionally, and always out loud. It's easy to fall into just skimming through it the way you might speed read a book, but doing so removes its power.

You can also record it on your smartphone, and even use editing software *(or hire someone on Fiverr.com)* to put some royalty-free, motivational music behind it. Then you can listen while you're driving, working out, at a boring lecture or work meeting, etc.

Some people also paste a copy of their "Big Why" in their cupboards or on their refrigerator where they'll see it each time they might otherwise reach for a snack. Still others ask their kids to help read it to them at breakfast or dinner.

You're only limited by your imagination. The point is, don't just write it down once and forget about it, make it something you're emotionally invested in every day. It really does make a difference!

Lastly, it's best to think of the "Big Why" as a kind of living document. Periodically, as you evolve and grow in your food journey, you'll want to revisit and redo the exercises, then revise your statement accordingly. This keeps it fresh and relevant. For this reason, it's also not something you need to get perfect on the first try. You can live with it for a little while and then revise it.

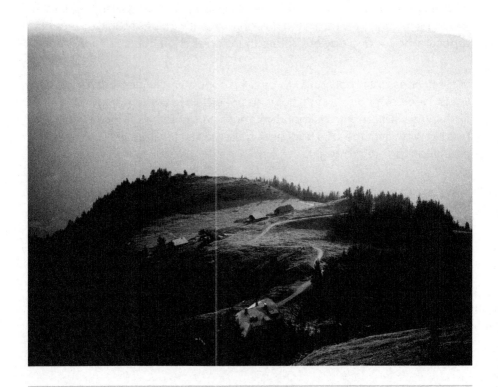

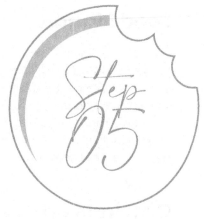

EXTINGUISH YOUR CRAVINGS

Overview

Did you know the same mechanism responsible for creating cravings also extinguishes them? That's why it makes no sense to say you are "broken" or "powerless." If you can develop cravings, you can extinguish them too!

The brain turns on a craving if it reliably leads to calories and nutrition but turns it off when it no longer does. It really is that simple, but most people unwittingly interfere with the process and perpetuate their cravings. In this chapter you'll see how to stop doing that.

I've written this chapter in plain English, and used stories for illustration, but if for any reason you feel reads too much like a science book, there's a clear summary of practical takeaways at the end.

Food Signals

Food signals initiate cravings. They can be external – like the colors on your favorite soda can, icons on a cereal box, or pictures of food on TV *(visual)*; sensations like heat and salty air at the beach *(physical)*; the lunchroom or your mother's house *(places)*; the smell of a pizza place or a bakery *(olfactory)*; the theme music of your favorite TV show *(auditory)*; or even the time of day. Food signals can also be internal – like feeling depressed or anxious – or physical experiences like being too hungry, full, cold, or tired.

Cravings are a sign of a healthy brain in action

In modern times, cravings are more easily attached to unhealthy foods because of the artificial concentration of calories and flavor, but they originally served a survival need – without them, we would have starved because we'd have lacked motivation to find and eat food. This is also why it takes longer to defeat cravings than it does to develop them. Once you've taught your brain a craving leads to a food reward, it thinks that craving is keeping you alive! And, because food was not nearly as abundant when the brain evolved, it's reluctant to give up this belief.

Dopamine regulates cravings in the brain. Higher levels are pleasurable, lower levels feel bad. The dopamine floods the brain in response to food signals, making you want to eat (Roitman et al. 2004). If you don't, dopamine levels drop precipitously, and you find yourself in a bad mood, which *also* makes you want to eat *(to relieve the associated discomfort)*.

Spot your favorite donut store sign ahead? Dopamine floods the brain to say, *"Oh boy, oh boy, go get some donuts and coffee!"* Pass it by without going in? Dopamine plummets as if to say, *"Go back and do it or I'll make you miserable!"*

These reactions are a 100% natural sign of a healthy brain doing its job. This is not to say you should just indulge, because the warped world we live in today will happily hijack your health for profit. An active defense is required, or the industry will siphon your life energy into its bank accounts. But **cravings – and**

all the bad feelings you get when trying to defeat them – are a normal and healthy function of the brain, not something to be ashamed of!

You're supposed to feel super excited when you eat in response to a previously rewarded food signal *(like the donut store sign),* and temporarily awful when you don't indulge. These intense feelings are due to normal dopamine shifts in the brain. As awful as they feel, they'll go away sooner than you think if you don't give in to them. You don't need to "do" anything about them, and there's nothing wrong with you for having them.

How your brain learns to find food

In early times food was scarce and we constantly had to lookout for new opportunities. For this reason, the brain values *new* sources of calories and nutrition more than existing ones and releases more dopamine in response. For example, the first time you go to your friend's house for their famous pasta dish, it's going to taste a lot better than the following week. You'll think more about getting invited back too. By the third or fourth time, it won't be nearly as pleasurable.

Watch out for delicious, new food experiences! If you unexpectedly encounter new, delicious food rich in calories, the ensuing dopamine hit may be strong enough to form a new habit from just that one experience. So, whenever you find yourself surprised by food pleasure, ask whether you want to crave it, and take steps to extinguish it right away if you don't!

About 20 years ago, my friend Hank told me a profoundly important anecdote. He was with his wife when he ordered a new dish at a diner. An almost insane amount of pleasure came over him when he took the first bite. He immediately put it down, looked at his wife and said, *"Oh, darling, I can't eat this, it's too good."* Apparently, he did this with some regularity. I don't think he knew the science because he wasn't that kind of guy, but he knew how quickly cravings formed and he didn't want this one. Hank's motto was: *"If it's too good, it's no good!"*

You can also use the phenomenon of immediate habit formation to your advantage. By seeking out delicious, new food experiences *within* the bounds of your food rules, you can train yourself to crave healthy food. There are hundreds of recipes on the internet, almost no matter what your dietary philosophy is. If you rotate enough new and delicious on-plan recipes into your life, you can quickly train your brain to crave healthy food!

Also, including enough variety ensures your brain won't get too "used to" any one dish and should continue to modestly raise dopamine levels at each meal to improve overall satisfaction levels *on* plan. You'll need a half dozen different, delicious, plan-compliant dishes to make this happen.

> **The next important thing to know about cravings is that new eating habits are automated quickly too.**

The brain is efficient. Because it believes food is scarce, it always wants to leverage new food sources once it's found them, so it's quick to hardwire cravings and habits, which lead to a reliable food reward on autopilot. This is why it sometimes *feels* like you can't remember passing the donut store sign, pulling into the parking lot, waiting in line, talking to the woman behind the counter, taking out the credit card, paying for the donuts, walking back to your car, opening the box, picking up a donut, and taking that first bite.

Cravings and habit automation are a priority until the reward becomes unavailable, or available only under certain specific circumstances. This is another reason it's important to interrupt undesirable habits before they form: Although you can extinguish virtually any unwanted behavior at any time, it's much less work – *and a lot less painful* – to prevent it from forming in the first place. You want to catch undesirable habit formation before the brain automates it.

Imagine it's 100,000 Years Ago

Suppose 100,000 years ago one of our ancestors *("Thag")* came across a chimpanzee who led him to an abundant banana tree. Thag's brain would quickly create a "follow-that-chimp" habit to find bananas more easily. The chimp would've become a food signal which triggered banana cravings and motivated Thag to follow.

Thag would've eaten as many bananas as he could when he found the tree, because food was scarce, and he wasn't sure where he'd find his next meal. It's unlikely Thag cared about portion control, body image, or how he looked in clothing. I'm pretty sure he didn't say, "Oy, Marta. Thag way too fat! Buffalo hide look awful on Thag. Thag hideous, Marta! Look away, Marta, look away!" No, Thag's main concern was survival, and that required eating as much as possible whenever he could.

Just like cravings are perfectly normal and natural, so, too, is the instinct to "consume mass quantities." It may not serve you well in today's food environment, but it's still a hardwired, healthy brain function. Therefore, feeling shame about appetite, obesity, and cravings is utterly incorrect. Let go of these pernicious thoughts and be proactive about which food signals you want to reinforce versus which ones you want to extinguish.

How the brain "unlearns" cravings

Please write this on the inside of your eyelids: "Cravings and habits are extinguished through discomfort." (*Don't really write inside your eyelids, I'm just emphasizing a point.*)

As per above, when a previously successful food signal stops leading to a reward, the brain protests by lowering dopamine levels, almost as if to say, *"Hey! What happened!? I could count on this signal in the past, so I'm not going to give up so easily! Let's see if I can make you miserable enough to reward me again."*

Remember our pasta friend? Suppose after enjoying pasta with him every Saturday for a month, out of the blue, one week he says he forgot to buy the ingredients. Your dopamine plummets, you feel sad, and start thinking about how to fix this awful problem. Maybe you can both go out and buy the ingredients together? Maybe he'll invite you over tomorrow instead? Maybe you could try to make it at home yourself.

The point is, you'd become psychologically uncomfortable, and would try to find an alternative way to acquire the dish. Getting it may even *seem* like the only way to dig yourself out of the sudden unhappiness you feel. That's just your brain protesting that its previously reliable signal *(your friend's house)* didn't lead to the reward. It's throwing a little temper tantrum.

I call this the "Where the f is my _ _ _ _!" reaction – as in, "Where the f is my pasta, chocolate, etc.!?" Knowing you'll experience this, removes the element of surprise and helps you power through something called the cravings extinction curve.

The Cravings extinction curve

In nature, it's unusual for reliable food signals to *suddenly* stop producing rewards. The chimp that Thag followed wouldn't have suddenly led him to completely empty trees. Instead, the trees would become gradually less productive, until, eventually, he encountered an empty one. Then, as more and more trees ran out of bananas, the habit would begin to *occasionally* fail. The previously reliable food sign *(the chimp)* would become less reliable, but still useful.

For this reason, Thag would not have given up the first time a chimp led him to a less productive or empty banana tree. Instead, he'd have doubled down and worked harder at following chimps, because finding bananas 80% of the time is much better than finding none at all. This was probably true even when his hit rate dropped a lot lower. In a very scarce food environment, even 20% success is better than nothing at all.

The brain seems to exaggerate cravings when a food signal begins to "dry up" and only produce rewards intermittently. In fact, it will as much as double the dopamine response. This is especially true if the reward occurs at *random* intervals, making it unpredictable and unexpected. That's why Thag worked twice as hard when the chimp signal began to fail. I call this the "slot machine effect." You become glued to the machine and keep pulling the arm because you never know when it's going to pay off. Intermittent, unpredictable rewards create *very* persistent behavior. *(The brain evaluates both the potential reward and the probability of obtaining it* (Schultz 2010).)

Indulging cravings at random produces more addictive dopamine patterns which are harder to extinguish. Your brain just "sits down at the slot machine" and keeps pulling the lever! (Kawa et al. (2019) *studied this same phenomenon in cocaine addiction and reported that intermittent, random access was, "...more effective at producing addictive behavior despite much less drug consumption." Intermittent, random availability of a reward is more powerfully addictive than higher volume!*)

This is why, if you don't want to give up a troublesome treat entirely, you should try binding it to a specific circumstance with a conditional rule. Perhaps you only eat bread with your spouse when dining out, and never more than two slices. Or maybe you only have coffee on Wednesday and Saturday afternoons within an hour of your workout, but no more than one cup. This way you eliminate the perception of an unpredictable, intermittent reward.

When you stop associating a food signal with a reliable reward, the brain enters an extinction curve for that habit. But before initiating a full extinction, it needs time to determine the reward has not become intermittently available at random. In other words, Thag's brain's first idea when the chimp led him to an empty banana tree was, "*Hmmmmmm... maybe just a few trees have run out of bananas; so, I'd better follow a lot more chimps to figure out if this is the case.*"

This is why the intensity of cravings does *not* drop in a downward sloping straight line when you first withdraw the reward from a signal. Instead, after a brief honeymoon period, you'll experience a sharp spike in cravings. Scientists call this an "extinction burst." *(I call it the "where the f is my _____!?" as per above.)*

Don't let this throw you! Just ride out the curve and don't indulge. You'll eventually move beyond the burst, and *then* your cravings can start their steady downward journey. Somewhere around the three-to-four-week range *(for previously daily habits)* the brain will have mostly given up and labeled the signal dormant. That's when your cravings become *much* more manageable in a more permanent way. You can expect to have only a few, much smaller spikes for a few weeks beyond this point before becoming almost entirely free of cravings in response to that particular signal.

PRACTICAL IMPLICATIONS

Summary

There are several critical takeaways from this scientific understanding of how cravings are extinguished.

First, watch out for delicious new experiences, especially if they're unexpected. Unexpected, new, and delicious are the perfect storm for developing a new craving fast! Whenever you have this experience, ask yourself if you want the craving and associated food habit. If not, immediately create a rule to avoid rewarding it again. Although you're armed with everything necessary to undo bad habits, it's much easier, and much less painful, to prevent them in the first place. *"If it's too good, it's no good."*

Second, remember you can extinguish any unwanted food habit! Identify the signal and remove the reward. If you don't want to give up the treat entirely, try binding it to a specific circumstance where it can't do too much damage. *"I only eat donuts on Sundays, no more than two, and only with my kids at the table."* Sometimes this works and sometimes it doesn't. Only you can determine whether it's worth the risk.

Third, expect a tantrum. *"Where the f is my _____!?"* Once you stop rewarding a craving, expect a brief honeymoon period followed by a *serious* spike in cravings and Pig Squeals. This is just your healthy brain doing its job. Prepare for it! Write your refutations. Read your Big Why. Have alternative plans instead of indulging. Consider eating a little extra healthy food during the tantrum phase, making your primary goal to power through the extinction curve rather than to lose weight that particular week. Work at actively turning off false emergency states during this time. Extinguishing a craving is a serious endeavor, so don't go into battle wearing a plastic helmet.

When cravings all but disappear during the initial honeymoon after removing the reward, some people think they're gone for good. They then understandably become frightened by the spike of the tantrum phase and think they must be doing something wrong. Extinction doesn't work this way. You must go through the full curve. The *only* way out is through. The tantrum will burn itself out sooner than you think if you don't reward it, even though your Pig says it will torture you forever. Don't give in! Your long-term freedom is worth the short-term pain! The worst is usually over in a few days.

Fourth, don't get cocky when cravings drop after the tantrum. When the tantrum is over and craving intensity drops again, some clients make a serious mistake. They become overconfident, think they've got it handled, and try a random indulgence to test this out. This not only immediately reactivates the craving but also labels it intermittent and random, making it twice as strong. It also resets the extinction curve to day zero! Just remember it will take several weeks beyond the tantrum before you can breathe a true sigh of relief.

Even when a craving is fully extinguished, it's still easy to reactivate addictive patterns if you bring back the reward. That's because extinguished cravings are never "erased" but simply labeled dormant. You can only get permanent relief by permanently decoupling the reward from the signal. Your brain will always have the predisposition to utilize the old pathway if you choose to reactivate it. Therefore, once you've extinguished a habit, don't revisit it! Re-establishing old cravings happens faster and easier than creating them in the first place, so once you've escaped cravings prison, don't go back to see your old friends.

Fifth, expect a few mini-tantrums toward the end of the month. These should be much easier to handle than the initial tantrum, but the same advice applies. It's your healthy brain doing its job again. Ride it out.

Sixth, because each extinction curve is attached to a specific food signal you may need to power through more than one curve to extinguish any given craving.

For example, Sally craves pizza whenever she passes a certain pizzeria on her drive home. She creates a rule to never buy pizza in person again, and successfully rides out the extinction curve without indulging. Thirty days later her drive home is free of pizza cravings. Has Sally eliminated them entirely?

Unfortunately, no.

Sally's brain *has* labeled pizzerias as a dormant signal, creating momentum, confidence, well-being, and probably some weight loss. But there could still be other active food signals for pizza. For example, Sally used to eat pizza with her dad every week at his apartment, but she hasn't seen him for a few months because she recently moved to a new city for work. When she finally does visit dad, Sally might have a pizza craving because she hasn't yet extinguished dad and his apartment as a signal for pizza. See what I mean?

Now, if Sally didn't understand how cravings worked, she'd think she failed and was doomed to be tortured with pizza cravings forever. But Sally did not fail! She *succeeded* in extinguishing the pizza-place-on-the-drive-home signal but had not yet addressed the pizza-at-her-dad's-place signal.

This is what I mean when I say that binging is not a unitary habit but a collection of habits.

At first, this may seem overwhelming. Your Pig will say, *"That's exhausting! You'll never extinguish all the signals for pizza or anything else because you're way too lazy. So just give up and stuff a slice or eight into your pie-hole, Okay? Yippee! Omnonmnomnom!"*

But the first extinction curve is usually the hardest to get through for any given craving, and the momentum created by succeeding helps you power through the rest. 80% of the problem is usually tied to one or two signals, with no more than a handful more for any given craving. So please don't let your Pig throw you. Remember, the majority of clients in my previous programs achieved an average 90% reduction in problem eating in just one month. They couldn't have done that if this were an impossible task.

The important takeaway is that not clearly understanding that more than one food signal can cause a particular craving can often cause people to give up thinking they've failed, when in fact they only had a little further to go to eliminate the craving. This is very sad because these individuals wind up perpetuating their cravings and feeling truly beaten down by them.

Seventh, plan to go through the whole curve from the outset. Tell yourself this is a serious endeavor that you should only have to ride out the extinction curve once for a given food signal. Make plans to support yourself through the entire process! Because your brain is a learning *and* unlearning machine, you can extinguish even the most brutally intense cravings in a relatively short period of time. You must, however, go through the curve completely. A lifetime of freedom is well worth the short-term pain, and the cost of an unwanted, life-long habit is infinitely worse. The only way out is through.

Eighth, extinction curves for less frequently occurring habits take longer to complete. For example, it's harder to extinguish a weekly pretzel and potato chips habit at your Saturday poker game than a daily chocolate habit. That's because, for weekly habits, you can only do the decoupling once every seven days, whereas you get seven opportunities per week for daily habits. But don't worry, I'll provide techniques to support you with less frequent habits in the next chapter. For now, just start extinguishing your unwanted daily habits, which constitute 80% to 90% of most people's food problems. Address all your unwanted daily habits and you'll feel 90% better right away.

Ninth, make a list of all your unwanted food signals prioritized in order of the damage they cause. Most of your cravings will be contained in the first few signals on this list, so the benefit of successfully extinguishing them should be monumental. Begin with the worst food signal and work your way down.

Finally, don't let your Pig derail you! Your Pig will say you must break your rules to escape the uncomfortable emotions associated with powering through an extinction curve, but these emotions result from a *temporary* dopamine dip which you don't need to do anything about. They'll pass sooner than you think. Tell your Pig you're willing to tolerate any level of discomfort to stick to your commitment.

To download a free copy of these practical takeaways, please visit www.DefeatYourCravings.com

AUTOMATE MOTIVATION AT THE MOMENT OF IMPULSE

If you've worked the previous steps, you're probably already experiencing some significant success. These are powerful methods indeed! But, if you're like most people, you're also encountering *occasional* troublesome food signals that you hadn't planned for.

You can address this by adjusting your food rules each time you encounter one. This process doesn't take as long as you think, and within five or six iterations you should feel that approximately 90% of your cravings are under control.

You can also brainstorm and come up with a long list of the different signals which *might* trigger a craving in the future, then adjust your rules and plans to cover them. In other words, be proactive, think through all the extinction curves you'll be facing – *especially those you don't encounter daily* – and ruthlessly attack them one by one.

Do what I've outlined above and you should start to encounter less trouble going forward.

There's actually one more tool you can use to not only nail the Pig's Cage shut but also make the whole experience more enjoyable, give you some protection for those inevitable encounters with unanticipated signals, and improve your level of food satisfaction.

What if you could arrange for your most powerful motivation *(and refutations)* to pop up automatically whenever you were about to eat *anything?* It only takes a little proactive work to substitute these reflexes for the Squeals the Pig wants you to listen to before meals. Plus, the technique in this chapter will provide you with a way to reinforce and remember all the other important insights you glean over the course of your work with the *Defeat Your Cravings* method.

This is a very exciting and powerful tool, but this step is also 100% optional. It's possible to extinguish your cravings without using this at all. Most people find it pleasurable and exciting once they learn to use this tool correctly, but some don't take to it and therefore don't use it. That's perfectly fine if that's you. However, I'd highly recommend you try it first before you decide because the results can be spectacular. No matter what you do, please don't let your decision about Step Six affect your implementation of the rest of the process.

Okay? Good! Let's go.

A concept from behavioral psychology called "Operant Conditioning" underlies this technique, so it's here I'll turn next.

OPERANT CONDITIONING

Operant conditioning is a simple concept with decades of science behind it. In a nutshell, when a behavior is followed by a reward, that behavior is more likely to recur.

For example, in my early 30s I had a 125-pound Doberman pincher named Dami. One day I was eating a piece of cheese by the refrigerator, and he happened to walk by and sneeze just before I gave him a nibble. You could see the wheels immediately turning in his head. "Hmmmmmm. Sneeze equals cheese?" He sat down in front of me, stared at me intently, and proceeded to sneeze again.

I thought that was super cool, so I gave him another piece. "Good boy, Dami. Good sneeze for cheese!" After that, he'd always run up to me at the refrigerator and sneeze for cheese. I'd inadvertently used operant conditioning to teach him that. I could've extinguished this behavior if I'd stopped giving him the cheese when he sneezed, but it was super cute, so I kept it going.

This is how the brain works. It's constantly monitoring our behavior and looking to reinforce anything that leads to calories, nutrition, and other vital resources.

Now, here's the thing: operant conditioning works for *thoughts,* too!

Remember I told you to be careful when thinking, "I'll just start again tomorrow," before you give in to a craving? That's because your brain will notice what you were *thinking* just before you "got the cheese." From its perspective, those thoughts might be part of what led to the food reward, so it'll try repeating them with increased vigor and frequency.

Our thoughts are conditioned by what comes immediately after you have them!

In the modern food environment, this principle tends to work against you because usually, when you encounter a food signal, the Pig provides an excuse to indulge, and you unwittingly reinforce that thought *(the Squeal)* if you give in. Indulging the craving makes the Squeal more likely to recur and harder to resist, whereas denying it does the opposite. The brain is always actively evaluating what leads to calorie acquisition and strengthening those neural pathways while weakening those pathways which don't.

The idea of the *Defeat Your Cravings Ritual* is to take control of what you think about immediately before you eat, then reinforce it meal after meal. Eventually whatever *you* want to think about starts to reflexively pop into your mind before you eat instead of the Pig's stupid excuses.

Let's get to it!

RITUAL PHASE ONE: INSERT A BRIEF PAUSE BEFORE YOU EAT

I recently had a little trouble with my eight-year-old cat Theo. And by a little trouble, I mean a *lot* of trouble. Out of nowhere he started throwing up several times per day, all over my apartment. I'd had a peaceful, easy time feeding him his whole life, but suddenly that was no longer the case.

The vet found nothing wrong. Theo didn't have diabetes, thyroid issues, liver problems, or any of the usual culprits. Frustrated – *and tired of living in a vomitorium* – I posted the problem on Facebook. I learned more about cats, cat food, and feline behavior than I thought any one person could possibly know, but nothing worked. Finally, one of my cat-loving friends asked me how quickly Theo ate.

"He's always eaten lightning fast," I told her. His fast-paced eating had never been a problem before, so I was skeptical this could be the issue. Apparently though, there's something in older cats called "scarf and barf." That's when the digestive system, which used to tolerate wolfing down food like a starving gorilla at an all-you-can-eat banana buffet, starts to age out of that tolerance.

I purchased a special bowl designed to slow him down, and it was a feline miracle. Problem solved.

After this, I got to thinking about how some clients had spontaneously taught themselves to use seven-eleven breaths not only before they did refutations, but also before meals. On average, they did better. I realized it wasn't solely because they were switching nervous systems, but because they were manufacturing some space to take control of their thoughts before eating. They'd learned to pause and think the things they *wanted* to think at mealtime. They didn't understand the supplemental benefit of reinforcing those thoughts with their food. In their minds they were just giving themselves the opportunity to eat more mindfully and with presence *(the opposite of "scarf and barf")*.

It turns out there are many helpful thoughts we can think about in that brief pause before eating, but if there is no space, there's no place to put them. If food reinforces the thoughts that come before it, you need to create enough space before eating to think desirable thoughts first.

Now, pausing in this way is *not* natural. Our instinct is to consume calories quickly before a competitor does. So, it's perfectly normal to feel resistant to this tool. I hope you'll power through and try it anyway.

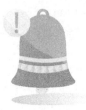

To begin, take one seven-eleven breath before you eat.

(Breathe in deeply for a count of seven, then out slowly for a count of eleven.)

Really, that's all.

Every time before you eat, pause long enough to take one deep, satisfying breath. Don't move on until you feel confident you can complete this 80% of the time. Allow one week, at minimum. Observe the impact. Do you eat more slowly? Feel more satisfied? Are you a little more present for your meal? Do you find yourself starting to feel a little calmer when you think about food?

Besides conditioning the mental pause muscle and creating the space to insert thoughts you wish to automate, the seven-eleven breath helps turn off any false alarms which might be firing in your reptilian brain. This makes the eating experience itself more peaceful and enjoyable. But that's not the primary goal, we're just building this to pause and be present.

Some people stop here and never move on to Phase Two of the Ritual. That's always an option. The difference between pausing and not pausing is night and day. It represents a critical difference in life philosophy. By inserting even the shortest pause before eating, you're affirming your desire to be proactive with your impulses and valuing the human ability to choose. It's the difference between who's in control – you or the Pig! This accomplishes a lot more than you think.

Some people also take a picture of their food before eating to create even more awareness and a visual food history.

RITUAL PHASE TWO: ADD A MANTRA

In your work so far, you've probably come across a few select refutations that have made a tremendous difference. Here you can shorten the best one to just a few words to say before eating.

For example, in case you can't tell, my Pig used to get me all the time with, *"It will be just as easy to start tomorrow."* My best refutation was: *"If I say 'just start again tomorrow' and indulge, I'll reinforce the craving and the thought, making it more likely I'll think the same thing and have a stronger craving tomorrow. So, it'll be harder to start again! When I'm in a hole, I must stop digging! I always use the present moment to be healthy."*

This is a bit long for the Ritual and would be annoying to have to read out loud three times per day, so I might extract only the conclusion of it to remind me of the sentiment: *"I always use the present moment to be healthy,"* or just, *"Eat healthy now!"*

It's easy to get excited and stuff long refutations (*and a bunch of other things*) into the pause, but people who do that often tire of the Ritual quickly and stop doing it.

Don't "stuff the Ritual" and burn out. Consistency is critical. Just like the "Big Why", this part of the method is much more like a vitamin than an antibiotic. You'll need to be able to do it even when you're in a foul mood with no motivation, not just when you're super motivated to defeat your cravings.

After reciting your mantra before meals for a few days you should find it starts to reflexively pop into your mind when you even begin to think about eating. That's the effect we're after. It'll be very weak and imperfect at first, but if you keep at it, you should notice a change after just a few days.

So, after you've become used to breathing before meals for a week or so, add a mantra. Live with this phase for at least a week as well. Build confidence in the process before moving on.

You don't have to go on to the next phase if you want to keep it simple. But for those of you who want more, you can enhance the power of the Ritual by adding the elements below.

RITUAL PHASE THREE: ADVANCED ADD-ONS

There are many more things you can insert once you start deriving real benefits from the Ritual. But please don't do this just for the sake of being a good student or "getting an A" in *Defeat Your Cravings*. Less is more, so if you ever find yourself feeling overwhelmed, remove something and shorten the work involved. *"When in doubt, leave it out!"*

Always protect your interest and commitment to using the Ritual consistently over trying to accomplish too much with it. The acid test is as follows; on a scale from one to ten *(where ten is highest)*, how much do you look forward to it? If the answer drops below a seven, you need to make your Ritual shorter or more relevant to your current struggles and goals.

In order of suggested attack, you can additionally insert the following into your Ritual: More breaths, more mantras, full refutations, portions of your Big Why, a "happiness dose" *(explained below)*, and inspirational quotes.

More Breaths

Within reason, the fact *that you pause* is more powerful than what you do with that pause. So, strengthen your pause muscle by adding one or two more seven-eleven breaths when you can. This is where you'll get the most bang for your buck.

More Mantras

The Pig almost never restricts itself to just one Squeal. For example, "start tomorrow" is often combined with "one bite won't hurt" as follows: *"One bite won't hurt – you can start your silly rules again tomorrow!"* So, in addition to, *"Eat healthy now,"* I could also add, *"One bite off plan is a tragedy,"* to bring up the sentiment of my best refutation, as in, *"Eat healthy now because one bite off the plan is a tragedy!"*

There's a place for full refutations in the Ritual, but short reminders are usually more effective. Develop the full refutation first, then abstract it to a few words which remind you of the main theme.

You'll find a full-page refutation for the "one bite" Pig Squeal in the Appendix. It includes ten reasons why one bite always hurts. The "one bite is a tragedy" mantra was abstracted from this full refutation.

Refutations

When a mantra isn't doing the trick, it's time to include a fuller version of the refutation. But remember, shorter is still better. Reading a long refutation at every meal gets old quickly.

How to condense it? There are several components in most effective refutations which correct the Pig's false logic, but usually only one which *really* hits the spot. That's the one to use. In the end you're not required to convince anyone but yourself; so if it works for you, use it.

When you place a refutation in the Ritual, you should always reference the Pig Squeal it addresses. This programs your mind to reflexively recall the refutation whenever the Squeal recurs.

For example, *"My Pig says it'll be just as easy to start again tomorrow, but if I indulge today, I'll be reinforcing both the craving and the 'start tomorrow' thought. Therefore, I must always use the present moment to be healthy."*

Or *"My Pig says one bite won't hurt, but it's never just a bite! One bite off plan is the difference between being my Pig's boss versus its bitch. One bite is a tragedy!"*

Read the above two examples and ensure you can identify the Squeal versus the refutation.

Try to avoid inserting more than three refutations in your Ritual even if your pause muscle has become very strong. Rituals quickly become "stale" and "boring" if the list gets too long. The only exception is for about 72 hours after making a serious mistake. During this recovery period it's important to include refutations for *all* the Squeals that bother you. More about this in Step Seven.

Big Why

You can also include elements of your "Big Why" in your Ritual.

If you do choose to incorporate parts of your "Big Why", make sure it's clear that sticking to the food plan is what will get you there. For example, *"Every time I deny the Pig and adhere to my food plan, I'm one step closer to being a healthy, confident, thin man who radiates a smiling presence!"* See how this works?

You can also add refutations. For example, after the above sentence you could add, *"My Pig says it's just as easy to start again tomorrow, but if I indulge today, I'll be reinforcing the craving and the 'start tomorrow' thought. Therefore, I always use the present moment to be healthy."*

Or you can incorporate multiple elements from the "Big Why." For example, *"Every time I deny the Pig and adhere to my food plan, I'm one step closer to being a healthy, confident, thin man who radiates a smiling presence, and is free from worry about heart attacks, strokes, diabetes, dementia, and cancer!"*

Or multiple elements from the Big Why *and* refutations.

Etc., etc., etc.

Next, you can add a gratefulness routine to provide a burst of automatic, happy feelings when you're about to eat. It also tends to make you happier overall.

Happiness Doses

Take a moment to ask yourself what you're happiest about today *because you've been complying with your food plan*. This serves several functions.

First, you'll get a little shot of dopamine when you think about denying the Pig's cravings. This is huge, because up until now I've been having you fight short-term pleasure from Slop with the long-term benefits in your Big Why. But programming yourself to feel immediately happy whenever you think about being on plan provides at least some *short-term* pleasure too. That's fighting fire with fire.

Second, pause to ask yourself what you're happiest about assigns your brain the task of finding things to be happy about. This stimulates the reticular activating system, the part of your brain that focuses your attention. It will start noticing happy moments more frequently throughout the day, which can make you a genuinely happier person overall.

If you'd like to use a happiness dose in your Ritual, just pause a little longer before eating and ask, "What am I happiest about, most content with, and/ or most grateful for because I am on my plan?"

For example, I recently realized staying on plan has made me confident taking off my shirt at the beach – something I would've never done before. My sister and brother-in-law recently visited me (*I live on the ocean*) and wanted to go for a swim. I didn't give it a second thought. I just took off my shirt and ran into the water! We swam together to the buoy about 100 yards out and back. It was invigorating. The feel of the water on our skin, the smell of the salty air, the sun on our backs, and the smiles on our faces. It was a great moment, iconic for the thrill I now feel just being alive.

See what I mean? By purposely recalling that moment of happiness just before eating and describing it with as many of my five senses as possible, I reinforced the feelings I wanted more of and associated them with the act of getting ready to eat. By doing this, I'm already feeling happy and much less tempted by Squeals and Slop.

Try to find something different to be happy about at each meal. At a minimum, describe the *same* happiness dose in a different way. A mentor once told me to walk around the same block 20 times and notice something different each time. I was amazed at how easy this was, and how for the rest of my day thereafter I kept noticing different things I hadn't observed before.

Sooner or later, your happiness doses will repeat no matter what, but see if you can get a dozen or so under your belt before that happens. Then, start asking yourself which one makes you happiest. Is there one thing which might be iconic for being happy in your life overall?

For example, after a year or so I discovered that although there were about 20 different things that were included as part of my happiness doses overall, feeling thin and moving more gracefully in yoga seemed to translate into happiness across my whole life. So, eventually, I just started recalling my last yoga practice and asking what new ways I experienced moving gracefully in my thin body.

Not everyone can find an iconic happiness moment. There's nothing wrong with you if one doesn't emerge. Just be aware it's possible, and perhaps you'll find it over time. Also, you don't need to practice yoga, that's just *my* center.

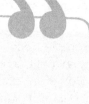

"To be yourself in a world that is constantly trying to make you something else is the greatest accomplishment."

Ralph Waldo Emerson

Lastly, doing your happiness dose in writing every time will probably take too long and cause you frustration. Instead, consider saying them out loud and, when you have the time, fully capture a few of them more in writing. Save those written happiness doses in a separate document that you can later access and read a few times per month.

Incorporating the happiness dose into your Ritual typically at least doubles the pause required before meals, so use it judiciously, and always monitor your willingness to keep doing the Ritual. Remember, it's better to shorten the Ritual than to start resenting it or skipping it entirely.

TYPICAL PROBLEMS WITH THE RITUAL

Hating Or Resenting The Ritual

I had a client who stopped performing the Ritual because, she said, *"It just doesn't seem right to pause and say all these things when there's a big steaming pile of food in front of me!"*

In retrospect, I wish I'd told her to dramatically shorten the Ritual, roll back one phase, or revert all the way to just one seven-eleven breath before eating. I also wish I had explained to her it's not *supposed to* feel right at first, just like stepping in the shower instead of going right to bed doesn't seem right when you begin. It's more natural to just eat the food or crash in bed. If you keep doing *only* what feels natural, it's unlikely anything will change.

In any case, if you're hating or resenting the Ritual, make it a whole lot easier by rolling back!

Forgetting It

When I first started using the Ritual, I found myself forgetting it with some frequency. I'd get angry with myself: *"Oh crap, I lost the opportunity to reinforce my favorite thoughts!"* But then I remembered the "consciously and purposefully" clause as it applied to food rules and began applying it to the Ritual too.

Occasionally forgetting is part of learning anything new. So, I set reminders for myself, and placed a little "Ritual statue" on my table. This was a $2 figurine I bought at a thrift store which I tried to look at only while reciting the Ritual before a meal. After doing that for a few days, seeing the figurine on my table reliably reminded me to perform the Ritual before eating. Problem solved.

Commit with perfection but forgive yourself with dignity, just like with your food rules. Excessive guilt is not permitted for missing part of your Ritual. So please don't stress it or I will have to send my Uncle Charlie to visit you. *(You won't like Uncle Charlie.)*

Also, performing the Ritual doesn't need to be a black-and-white thing, where you either do it in its entirety or skip it. Instead, you can have longer and shorter versions to use as circumstances allow. Sometimes you can also perform the Ritual in your head instead of out loud. Perhaps you recite the full version out loud before breakfast, then recite a shorter version in your head for lunch and dinner.

You'll get the best impact by reading the Ritual out loud, slowly and purposefully, and the full version will have more of an impact than the shorter one. But think of it like going to the gym: Sometimes you've got it in you to do a super-intense workout, but other times it's all you can do to show up and walk slowly on the treadmill for a few minutes. Getting your butt to the gym and exercising even just a little bit is still infinitely better than blowing off your workout entirely.

The idea is to show up consistently, regardless of how intense a "workout" *(Ritual)* you're up for doing at any given time. Sometimes showing up can be as easy as just taking one seven-eleven breath at any given meal.

In other words, you've got options!

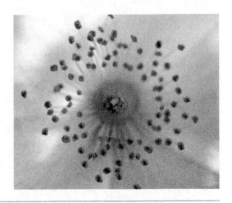

Difficulty Doing It Around Others

The above principles doubly apply when dining with others. Doing the Ritual slowly and purposefully out loud before eating is not always possible with others at the table. You could excuse yourself to the bathroom and do it there, or just use a shortened version in your head. You could just do one mantra or seven-eleven breath and nothing else. Remember, the difference between pausing and not pausing is monumental.

Also, you can skip any given meal if you need to. I promise, no *Defeat Your Cravings* police will come arrest you.

"What are you in for?"

"I didn't do my Ritual!"

That's not a conversation you'll be having any time soon, I promise!

All kidding aside, understand the principles behind what makes the Ritual more versus less effective, then just keep striving toward them. I've found those who use it *in any form* before at least 50% of their meals get the best results. That seems to be the inflection point. Also, please remember, lots of people recover without doing the Ritual at all.

If you're going to perform the Ritual, aim to do it with at least half of your meals. But rather than beating yourself up or fighting with yourself to get there, if you find the Ritual difficult to perform consistently it might just be a sign you need to rework it a bit. Perhaps it's too long *(the most common problem)*, contains something you don't fully believe, or needs to be infused with something more motivating and personally exciting. Evaluate and adjust until it seems easy again.

Eventually your Ritual should become something you look forward to, not viewed as a chore or obligation. For the Ritual to function optimally you'll want to make it something you "get to" do, not something you "have to" do.

Kids Won't Let You DO IT

Some people create a game or a "Ritual song" and recruit their kids to do it along with them. Others run off to the bathroom and lock the door for a few minutes, excusing themselves to go wash their hands. Others recite it in their head. Still others ask their spouse or parents to help out with the kids so they can steal away for a few minutes break to perform the Ritual before meals. Where there's a will, there's a way!

Not Having Enough Time

As per above, make sure to create shorter versions of your Ritual and alternate between reading it out loud and in your head. Reciting it out loud engages the brain more fully so that the learning process is both stronger and faster, but there's still much good value in saying it softly in your head. Every meal is a brain-programming opportunity! Just do your best to leverage this to whatever extent you can.

Even Olympic athletes don't work out full force every single time they go to the gym. They take time off when needed. You too can vary the energy, frequency, and intensity with which you conduct the Ritual. Just find a rhythm that works for you.

Seems Meaningless After Giving Into Cravings

If doing your Ritual seems meaningless after breaking your rules and there's a voice in your head that says, *"This is bulls---t,"* you'll want to put it aside for 72 hours and use the special Recovery Ritual I'll highlight in the next chapter instead. Except for the pause, the Ritual will indeed seem meaningless and stupid after a serious mistake. It's better to change it to something you can believe in for a few days than to force yourself through it when you don't.

Integrating It With Prayer, etc.

Some religions already include a Ritual by gathering together in prayer before meals. If this is your practice, adding an opportunity to reflect about why you're happy about staying on plan, like including a mantra to encourage adherence to your rules, is a great way to attach the *Defeat Your Cravings* habit to something you're already doing. The goal is not to replace prayer but to enhance it.

Why Go Beyond the Seven-Eleven Breath at All?

Finally, some people ask, *"If using a simple seven-eleven breath makes such a big difference, then why complicate the Ritual any further with mantras, refutations, and parts of your 'Big Why,' etc.?"*

For starters, breathing deeply *does* indeed make a big difference. It slows you down, teaches you to pause and to be more mindful before eating, and it gives you the opportunity to make better food choices. What it *doesn't* do is reinforce the thoughts you want to have about food instead of entertaining Pig Squeals. It also doesn't reinforce your specific motivation to stick to your Food Rules. Lastly, it doesn't reinforce the refutations that strengthen your resolve to Cage the Pig.

DEALING WITH INFREQUENT FOOD SIGNALS

Remember, overeating is a collection of habits, not a unitary habit. Any given craving is usually attached to more than one food signal, and the ones which occur less frequently often surprise us. Often when people encounter these signals and suddenly feel a craving again, they give in and feel like the method as a whole "isn't working." However, a much more accurate assessment is that they've succeeded with daily triggers but failed to plan for less frequent ones.

For example, it took me a very long time to give up chocolate completely once I decided to adopt the rule. I'd be largely successful for months at a time, which really improved my *day-to-day* life, but I kept encountering infrequent situations that would stimulate overwhelming cravings.

You know those chocolate bunnies you see around Easter time? OMG! Also, at Halloween, my mom would have boxes of Malomars *(chocolate covered marshmallow cookies)* laying around. At Thanksgiving, my sister would make chocolate chip cookies to die for!

Now, here's the problem. It takes 21 to 30 extinction exposures to complete an extinction curve. *(An extinction exposure is when you're exposed to the signal but don't reward the ensuing craving.)*

Unfortunately, holiday food signals only come around once per year. That means these extinction opportunities are few and far between. So, for a while, I was still indulging in little chocolate binges a few times per year. Although these infrequent binges were still much better than my former cravings-tortured daily life, it was a residual problem which took way too long to beat. I could have suffered far less if I'd known the simple technique I'm about to share.

I eventually achieved full compliance by refuting the Pig after each Holiday mistake – postmortem. Today, though, I know a much better way. Schedule an email to yourself to arrive just before, during, and after each of these events to remind you of anything you want to be forefront in your mind. You can also use simple smart phone reminders as well.

Although I had many tools at my disposal, including the ones I've highlighted so far:

- ☑ Separation.
- ☑ Refutation.
- ☑ Turning off false alarms.
- ☑ The "Big Why."
- ☑ Understanding the science of food cravings and how they are extinguished.
- ☑ The Ritual.

Yet before using this scheduling technique I didn't know how to get myself to focus on them during these infrequent bingeing events.

In virtually every email system there's a function that allows you to queue your message up to send later. In Gmail, there's a little arrow next to the send button that lets you do this. You can search YouTube.com to learn how to do it in other email systems. And virtually every smart phone has a handy reminder app. And you know what? Even an old-fashioned paper and folders tickler system will let you program reminders to arrive just in time! Any of these systems can be extremely helpful for infrequent food signals.

If I were still struggling with how to deal with chocolate on Easter, Thanksgiving, and Halloween, for example, I could write a refutation for the Squeals I'd anticipate hearing as the events grew near, and schedule them to show up a day or two before each one.

I might also include relevant portions of my "Big Why," inspirational pictures, quotes, videos, music, etc.

I could even attach a different version of my Ritual to use that week to include the most relevant refutation.

I might also add a description of the healthy treat I planned to eat *instead* of the chocolate chip cookies I'd be tempted to eat on Thanksgiving, or the Malomars on Halloween, etc.

I might remind myself where the produce store was on the way to Thanksgiving dinner so I could buy a bunch of fruit to bring over. Etc.

The point is you can head off trouble at the pass by simply being proactive. Just think through a series of reminders that come from your higher self to help you successfully confront the anticipated-but-infrequent signals that await.

Choose the subject line for each reminder carefully. It must get your attention amid a sea of day-to-day emails, spam, etc. For example, "Thanksgiving reminder" is much less effective than "WARNING: Cookies are a Gateway to Your Downward Spiral or Personal Hell!" See what I mean?

It's best to schedule something before, during, and after the anticipated problem. Don't assume you're safe after the event has passed. A lot of people require extra support for a day or two after the event has occurred. This doesn't mean you'll always use exactly three reminders. For example, the chocolate Easter bunnies are around for a week or two, before and after Easter, so I'd need several reminders throughout the season. Sometimes you'll also need support throughout the day, especially at large family and social gatherings.

With these proactive techniques in hand to help you maintain your motivation in the face of added societal pressures and get your higher self to show up at the moment of temptation and deal with infrequent food signals, you now have everything you need to extinguish your cravings except *(please cover your Pig's eyes while you read the next three words.)* A recovery plan!

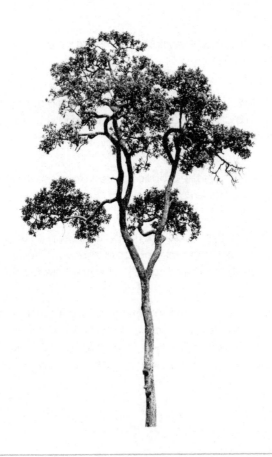

　　　　　　　ENHANCING AND SPEEDING UP THE PROCESS

HAVE A
RECOVERY PLAN

"Success is not final, and failure is not fatal. What counts is the courage to continue."

Winston Churchill

Always tell the Pig you'll never make another mistake again, no matter how many missteps you've made in the past. That's because any other attitude invites the Pig to incessantly bother you until you give in. Committing with perfection when aiming at the target is the *only* way! The Pig must believe the rules are set in stone, and know that you're resolute about following them perfectly, forever.

However, most people do make mistakes. We fall down and get up again until we can stay up for good. That's how the process—*and progress*—works.

For this reason, it's important to not only know how to forgive yourself with dignity after you've made a mistake, analyzed it, and incorporated the necessary adjustments, but to also have a specific recovery plan in place.

Don't skip this step please, no matter how well you're doing. Having a recovery plan in place is critical.

THE MOST IMPORTANT THINGS TO KNOW ABOUT RECOVERY

There are several critical things to know about recovery that can make all the difference. Most people get these wrong and unwittingly prolong their suffering.

First, recover from an overeating episode with a week of normal eating, not by restricting your calories, over-exercising, or engaging in any other compensatory behavior. Crazy eating is balanced by normal eating, *not* with more crazy eating! Attempting to compensate keeps you on the feast-and-famine roller coaster, exacerbates false alarms, and aggravates your urges.

Second, after a mistake, if there's no medical reason you can't consume fresh, tender, leafy greens, throw a half pound in a blender with two cups of water and drink it down. This helps the Slop go through faster. It also reassures your survival drive that nutritious, healthy food *is* available despite the recent intake of junk. This, in turn, reduces cravings for *more* Slop.

Third, you'll inevitably have significant feelings of disappointment, hopelessness, helplessness, and self-criticism after a serious eating mistake, especially if it's the first one you've made in a long time. You'll probably feel you've lost your motivation. You'll question whether this method works. It will seem too difficult, and you'll start wondering what else you might try instead. These feelings result from the dramatic dopamine crash that occurs after the

Pig Party is over. Don't take it seriously.

See, the Pig is very excited about the Slop you fed it, and thinks your rules no longer apply. It knows your rational thinking has been temporarily rendered less available by the indulgence and will pull out all the stops to take advantage of this weakened state.

Just as with strong cravings, however, it's *not* a sign there's anything wrong with you! Analyze what caused the mistake and make any necessary adjustments to your rules, ritual, and plans. Then simply just move on.

Once you've converted guilt into responsibility, forgive yourself with dignity. Remind yourself nobody's perfect. Absolutely every successful client I've ever known has made numerous serious mistakes along the way. I have too.

Also, don't fall for the Pig's ridiculous Squeal that says, *"You're not perfect, therefore you're nothing, so you should just give up and binge more. Yippee, let's do it now!"*

That is just another pathetic attempt by the Pig to get more Slop. You're *not* damaged goods! Don't let the Pig convince you otherwise.

Finally, if this the first mistake you've made in a long time, the Slop will have been *very* unexpected and therefore will have created an exceptionally large dopamine release. Unfortunately, this means the ensuing crash will be even greater, and you'll find yourself in a much worse mood than you've experienced for a long time. The only way to overcome this is to eat normally and go through it. You'll feel much better within 72 hours if you don't feed the Pig anymore!

All these negative thoughts and bad feelings are inevitable, especially if you were doing well for an extended period of time before the mistake. You don't need to do anything about them.

Fourth, remind yourself the key to success is to get back up and resume quickly, then learn as much as you can from the experience. Successful people have the *most* failures behind them because they've learned from every mistake. *"The name of the game is staying in the game until you win the game."* That's probably my most favorite line I've ever said! Resolve to learn everything you can from every mistake. If you missed the bullseye, ask yourself why? By how much? In what direction? Get up, adjust your aim, and shoot at the target again.

Fifth, act more superior to your Pig than usual. This really counts! If you find yourself thinking, *"I don't care, I just want more,"* actively change your internal dialogue to, *"I don't care that you don't care, Pig! I know you want more, but I'm going to stick to my rules forever. Too bad, so sad. Now go back to your cage!"* Make the Pig fear you like a wolf pack fears the alpha wolf.

After a mistake, when you find yourself feeling disconnected, having trouble concentrating, or just don't quite feel like yourself, say, *"Hey Pig! I know you're clouding my thinking in hopes I won't be able to reason my way to good food choices. I won't have it!"*

Sixth, write down and refute all the Squeals which bother you. The Pig's arguments will mostly be centered around keeping the episode going so you can indulge more, but some of the Squeals will also be about your character. It will say how weak, powerless, and pathetic you are for having made the mistake, etc. Refute like never before!

Below are a few power-refutations for common post-binge Squeals curated over many years.

Post-Binge Squeal #1: "You're powerless to stop overeating. It's hopeless."

The illusion of powerlessness is the cardinal sin in overeating – the psychological cancer upon which all other Pig Squeals rely. Work hard to develop your own refutation for it and put it in your Ritual *(if you use one)* for 72 hours after a serious mistake. This might do more for you than anything else in this book. I finally overcame the powerless Squeal for good when I wrote a refutation which emphasized all the evidence of success I could muster. I took special care to be accurate so the Pig couldn't poke holes in it:

"I've eaten 94% of my meals on plan for years, and maintained my exercise, produce intake, and weight within 7% of my ideal. I'm a healthy person who largely acts with integrity when it comes to his values and goals. I am far from powerless. The more I flex my 'binge-free muscle' now the stronger it gets, and the more permanently binge-free I become. If the Pig says, 'Just one more day of binging,' I say. 'Just one more day of healthy eating,' instead. I forgive myself for absolutely everything."

Your numbers will be different, but even if you've only eaten 20% of your meals on plan for a few years, this is still a powerful refutation against powerlessness because someone who was a powerless person would eat 100% of their meals off plan. So, just make a conservative estimate you believe to be true.

Overcoming these Squeals is also much easier if you can shift to what psychologist Martin Seligman identifies as an "optimistic explanatory style." (Seligman 2006) For example, an optimist might interpret a serious food mistake as a temporary divergence from their plan due to a specific, unexpected food-signal: *"This was a surprisingly stressful week at work which stimulated chocolate cravings I wasn't prepared for;"* whereas a pessimist might say, *"I'm a pathetic loser and powerless over chocolate. It's hopeless."*

Watch out for pessimistic, character-based, insulting explanations. Teach yourself to adopt an optimistic style. Self-compassion researcher Dr. Kristen Neff says to talk to yourself as if you were talking to a good friend, be compassionate and kind to yourself.

Finally, try this thought experiment. Suppose an evil dictator kidnapped the person or pet you most love or admire in this world. It could even be a public figure or celebrity who really inspires you. Now, assume the dictator says he'll treat this person kindly provided you comply 100% with the food rule you just broke for a full year. However, if you break it again, they'll place this person in the dungeon and torture them daily for the rest of their life. Would you break the rule again?

Of course not! That's because you aren't powerless, and the prospect of someone you care about being tortured every day isn't worth th e short-term pleasure of the rule break. It's just a matter of priorities. The Pig is an evil dictator, and *You* will feel tortured every day if you keep breaking your plan. You're not powerless, so stop letting the Pig make you think you are.

Post-Binge Squeal #2: "More Slop will make you feel better."

This Squeal usually only occurs after a serious mistake the Pig convinced you to make. If it hadn't done so, you wouldn't need to feel better in the first place! It's the dopamine crash that makes you feel so badly, but eating more Slop will only make it worse. Also, try to remember that an additional overeating episode after a mistake will not make you feel as good as the first one because it won't be *unexpected*. The dopamine hit won't be nearly as strong, and the foul mood will return more quickly. The only way to restore your normal sense of balance and well-being is to ride out the bad feelings until they pass.

Post-Binge Squeal #3: "Screw it, you already blew it, so keep going!"

While the "start again tomorrow" and "just one bite" lies are responsible for *beginning* more overeating episodes than any other Pig Squeal I've seen, the "screw it you already blew it" Squeal causes the most damage. It turns simple slips into all-out food orgies, which really sap people's confidence. Fortunately, there are several very good ways to combat it.

First, acknowledge that every moment is an opportunity for harm reduction. Five cupcakes are better than 15! One whole pizza is better than two. Six thousand extra calories does twice the damage of 3,000, etc. Every bite counts, every last one!

Second, making a mistake does *not* compel you to compound and multiply it! If you accidentally run a red traffic light, are you obligated to run the remaining ones within a five-mile radius? If you chip a tooth, are you compelled to go get a hammer and bang the rest out? If you slip and fall while hiking, are you obligated to roll down the mountain to the bottom? If you touch a hot stove, do you immediately think, *"Well, now I have to do that a whole bunch more times?"* Of course not!

Third, remember: *"If you're not perfect then you're nothing!"* is a big hairy Pig lie. If you make a mistake you're not supposed to say, *"I'm pathetic. Obviously, I can't resist making more!"* Instead, figure out what went wrong and use it to make course corrections as required.

Then, collect evidence of success. Maybe you ate half the cake instead of the whole thing? Great! Perhaps the episode lasted for a few hours instead of a few days? Fantastic. Identify how things are improving and figure out how to leverage that learning next time. Collecting evidence of small successes causes the gradual buildup of a success identity, which increases confidence and helps you to stay on plan longer.

After you've figured out what went wrong, forgive yourself with dignity, get up, and aim at the bullseye *again*. Successes are just people who fell and got up more times than failures did. Human beings are learning machines. Human neurology is set up to glean as much useful information as possible from every mistake. As a result, you'll almost always get better if you keep aiming at the bullseye, examining why you missed it, and adjust accordingly.

Fourth, what might successful people you admire do in this situation? For example, when Hussein Bolt trips and falls while practicing for a race, does he have a tantrum, start throwing his shoes everywhere, and say "screw it?" Not quite.

Finally, remember your Pig doesn't have a time machine and can't possibly know what you'll eat tomorrow. But you can *always* know what you'll eat in the present moment. The only time you can put food in your mouth is in the present, and it's *always* the present. Therefore, you can be assured of eating healthy forever if you always use the present moment to eat healthily. It doesn't matter what you did five hours, five minutes, or even five seconds ago. It doesn't even matter if you're indulging your cravings as you read this sentence. Once you stop breaking your plan *now*, you win! So just tell yourself, *"I never break my rules now!"* and you'll be fine.

Post-Binge Squeal #4: "You deserve it."

Focus on what you *really* deserve, like the items listed in your "Big Why." For example, I deserve to feel like a tall, thin leader in the world, free from worries about strokes, heart attacks, kidney disease, and diabetes. I deserve to feel confident in myself, to live in full integrity with my values, and feel confident in my body.

Overeating, beginning with "one more little treat," takes away most of these feelings immediately. Taking one step further off plan after a mistake makes you naturally begin to think, *"How much can I get away with? How will I hide the evidence? How will I make up for it later? When can I sleep it off? How do I avoid being seen?"* This is not a reward, it's torture, and you certainly don't deserve that.

For me, a reward is going for a walk on the beach, in the mountains, around the lake, or in the forest. It's taking a nap, reading a book, practicing some yoga, talking to a friend, do some writing or journaling, work on something interesting, listen to an inspiring podcast, improvising on the piano, jumping in the pool or the ocean, call my niece or my nephew, take a psychology course, cuddle with my super-annoying-but-very-lovable cat, going to the movies, strolling on the pier, singing in the shower, planning my next accomplishment, thinking about my next vacation, listening to a course on tape, turning on some music, watching a great movie, binge watching something on Netflix, etc.

A brief sugar high, followed by days of misery is not a reward, it's a punishment!

Seventh, have a recovery meal plan at the ready. Overeating episodes tend to cycle downward when left to their own accord. The post-indulgence dopamine crash is very uncomfortable, so it's common to seek out another indulgence for short-term relief. People also tend to panic about weight gain from the mistake and attempt to compensate by over-restricting. That keeps you in feast-and-famine mode and aggravates cravings. Finally, blood sugar is destabilized by all the sugary, rich food you probably ate when you indulged, and it's natural for the brain to seek more sugar to compensate. All in all, it's a perfect storm.

You can fix this with a recovery meal plan that is *not* geared toward weight loss and focused on lower-glycemic, filling foods. Aim only to maintain your weight for 72 hours while allowing your dopamine and blood sugar levels to re-stabilize. A normal, healthy, and substantial meal plan will make you feel immensely better in record time. Every other option just keeps the dopamine and blood sugar roller coaster going, aggravating cravings and discomfort.

Now, please cover your Pig's eyes while you read this next paragraph.

It's useful to develop a specific recovery meal plan while you're *on*-plan and have your wits about you. It should cover a 72-hour period, and not include any high-glycemic, sugary foods. Sugar, flour, white potatoes, dried fruit, alcohol, etc., should be completely off limits for this three-day period when you'll aim to recover your food sanity.

Assuming your doctor doesn't object, focus on filling, satisfying meals like beans and greens if you're plant-based, or protein and greens if you're not. I'd also suggest you consume three meals and two light snacks per day during this period so you can avoid any dramatic caloric hits. Remember, the goal is to even out and restore your blood sugar and dopamine levels.

Eighth, switch to a special Recovery Ritual for 72 hours (if you're using the Ritual at all). The normal Ritual will be ineffective for a few days after an overeating episode because your Pig's voice will be screaming, *"You just proved this to be B.S. by making a serious eating mistake!"* in the background. Until you're solidly back on track, this Squeal will unfortunately sound true. Also, the Pig Squeals you hear will be different during the recovery period – they'll focus much more on weakening your character, calling you powerless and pathetic, so you'll need a different set of refutations to handle these.

Therefore, during the recovery period, adapt your Ritual to help with short-term focus and motivation rather than reinforcing long-term goals, etc. Focusing on long-term goals at a time when you're not capable of believing them is anti-motivating and depressing. Your goals will still be there in a few days after you've recovered, I promise. Until you're solidly back on track, the ideal strategy is to focus on short-term commitments and actions that will make you feel better immediately.

For example, you might use the following commitment statement to begin your Recovery Ritual:

"I commit to eating ALL my meals and snacks, and not trying to lose any weight at all until <insert date and time representing 72 hours since your last serious eating mistake>. I will not over-restrict in any way and will resist the urge to overeat no matter how awful this feels. I know I'll feel much better when I'm back to my normal, cravings-free life in just a few days, but the only way out is through."

You also might consider adding a few progress-related prompts to your Recovery Ritual for motivation to pull you through this period. *"How many* hours have passed since my serious eating mistake?" "What benefits am I experiencing because I am 100% on plan since then?" "Is my digestion better?" "Do I feel less bloated?" "Am I experiencing fewer aches and pains?" "Do I look less puffy?" "Am I getting back to my normal, productive self?" "Am I better able to connect with others?" "Is my thinking starting to return to positive?"

For about 72 hours after the episode, you can add refutations for *all* the Squeals that might be bothering you. It's likely that at least one of the post-binge Squeals discussed above will be useful.

Finally, you can end your Recovery Ritual by saying, *"It's almost <insert day plus one> days already!"* Be sure to add the "plus one" to your day count. For example, for the 24 hours after your last eating mistake you can say, *"It's almost Day Two already!"*

I know this seems weird, but it really helps pull you through. The reason is, most people absolutely despise the first day after an episode because everything feels so crappy, and the Pig will beat you down about this to take advantage. *"OMG, another Day One? Are you ever going to learn? Just give up already and binge your face off!"* By starting out saying, *"It's almost Day Two already!"* you shift the focus and give yourself strength. You feel hopeful and enthusiastic. Besides, you're not lying because you said "almost." Day One is, in fact, almost Day Two! Remember, the Pig can't put you on the stand in court. You're not going to have to swear an oath to tell the truth, the whole truth, and nothing but the truth. So, lie to the Pig to take away its power!

Once you're back on track for 72 hours, go back to your regular Ritual. It's too much work to keep up the Recovery Ritual forever, and many of the thoughts and feelings that were bothering you immediately after the overeating episode should have faded by then.

Lastly, you might want to consider writing a Recovery Ritual even if you don't use the Ritual during normal, day to day life. It's a powerful tool that can make the 72 hours after a serious indulgence much more bearable and more importantly, should help make it much easier to get back on track.

To download a free one-page cheat sheet on the key items in the recovery process, please visit www.DefeatYourCravings.com

BUILD COMMUNITY SUPPORT

In my original book, I railed against the notion of using dependency to overcome overeating. I wanted to challenge the predominant thinking in our culture that emphasizes "powerlessness" over cravings, the inability to overcome them on your own, the need for sponsors and perpetual accountability. I felt these notions contributed greatly to the many years I spent suffering from overeating and thought everyone should just recover on their own. After all, that's how I did it, all by my lonesome!

Despite this, I was flooded with requests for group and individual coaching, accountability, and a community of like-minded peers. Eventually I gave in and started a small program. And while it took me almost eight years to fully defeat my cravings and recover from overeating on my own, individuals we were coaching did so in just a few months. Keep in mind, not all of them achieved this, but the majority who took the program seriously certainly made significant progress *much* faster than I had.

I know it sounds weird, because who wouldn't want to have a coaching program flooded with clients, but I still wanted to be sure I was doing the right thing in continuing to offer such a program. So, I decided to dig into the research on group interventions to see if there was scientific research to support it. Indeed, there was:

- ☑ A highly cited study in the New England Journal of Medicine (Wadden et al. 2005) reported that adding a group intervention resulted in 81% more weight loss at the one-year mark as compared to other interventions *(26.7 versus 14.7 pounds)*.

- ☑ A meta-analysis of 27 randomized, controlled studies with 1,853 participants published in the *International Journal of Eating Disorders* (Grenon et al. 2017) concluded group intervention was significantly more effective at getting people to stop binge eating. This was true both for complete abstinence as well as decreased frequency.

- ☑ A study in *Diabetes,* the journal of the *American Diabetes Association,* which publishes research on physiology and pathophysiology of diabetes mellitus, conducted a randomized, controlled weight loss trial with 257 people and concluded that, "...group intervention may be more effective than solo contact in achieving dietary and activity changes associated with weight loss." Group participants enjoyed significantly longer improvements, whereas the impact of solo interventions seem to have disappeared by the two-year mark (Trief et al. 2018).

- ☑ A six-month randomized controlled trial conducted at Mito Kyodo General Hospital in Japan with 188 overweight adults was reported in the journal *Obesity Facts*. **More than double the weight loss was observed for those who received group support versus education alone** (Nakata et al. 2011). This was of particular interest to me since I needed to know whether group support was warranted over and above the book alone.

- ☑ A study in the *Journal of Consulting and Clinical Psychology* (Renjilian et al. 2001) concluded, "Group therapy produces greater weight loss than individual therapy, even among those clients who express a preference for individual treatment." What's fascinating here is that regardless of what the person *thought* was better for them, and which mode *they* were more comfortable with, group intervention outperformed individual treatment on both BMI and average weight loss.

- ☑ For more serious weight struggles, a study on 78 bariatric surgery patients *(published in the official journal of the American Society for*

Bariatric Surgery) found significantly more weight loss twelve months post op for those who attended more than five weekly support groups versus those who attended five or less.

☑ And, if your Pig tortures you about previously failed weight loss attempts? This study on the effectiveness of group interventions reported in the *Journal of Health Psychology* should pique your interest. Latner and Ciao (2014) found that a greater number of past weight loss failures independently predicted *more* weight loss in a group environment.

☑ A handful of other studies documented more weight loss in groups, but in smaller amounts. For example, the *Journal Metabolic Syndrome and Related Disorders* published a study (Miller et al. 2009) citing 22.6% more weight loss in groups. I won't review all such studies here.

☑ A pair of prominent professors at Harvard also highlight the importance of your social circle in determining obesity in their book *Thinfluence*. Dr. Walter Willett, professor of epidemiology and nutrition, and Malissa Wood, assistant professor of clinical medicine, point out that the chance of obesity increases by 57% if your friends are obese. Comparable percentages for siblings and spouse are closer to 40%, which suggests the people you choose to associate with have significantly more influence than your spouse or family. Clearly there's an opportunity to improve through consciously developing a social circle with similar values and goals around weight and food behavior.

There was plenty more research, but since this book isn't a research review but rather a practical guide to defeating your cravings, I did not include more references here. Suffice it to say I believe the preponderance of the evidence strongly supports the idea of helping people defeat their cravings in a group environment.

I think there's another reason our group coaching programs worked so well. I was lucky enough to trade consultations with Dr. Stephen Covey *(educator, businessman, and author of the immensely popular "The 7 Habits of Highly Successful People")* in 2002. I was seeking leadership advice and he suggested I recruit and train leaders who could cultivate something he called "interdependence." Dr. Covey saw development as going from *dependence, as in,* "I need you or I'll fail – I can't do it myself," to *independence, as in,* "I can do it all by myself," to *interdependence, as in,* "I don't *need* to be part of a team; I *want* to be part of a team, because we can accomplish more together than I can on my own."

In my previous book, I helped move my clients from dependence *(requiring the use of sponsors and accountability to defeat their cravings, etc.)* to independence *(the ability to stop overeating on their own)*, but did not guide them to interdependence. The group program, in contrast, lets people leverage a team to recover faster, stronger, and more permanently. In other words, the book made them independent but the community created interdependence.

Also, a big part of the Pig's power is its ability to make people feel like they are different and broken. Most people think nobody else struggles the same way they do, so there must be something wrong with them. I know it sounds crazy to think you're alone in this struggle when fully 40% of the population is obese, but overeaters really do feel this way. Connecting with a community helps dissolve this notion. You'll see that other people have Pigs that Squeal in very similar ways to your own. You'll hear them struggling with similar emotions and thoughts, and you'll feel infinitely less alone.

Watching approximately 2,000 people go through our program of groups, individual coaching, and accountability also showed me that joining a group of like-minded people can help in the following ways:

- ☑ Overcoming sticking points.
- ☑ Identifying Squeals that some individuals might have trouble hearing on their own.
- ☑ Bolstering motivation and determination to cage the Pig.
- ☑ Brainstorming potential food rule revisions.
- ☑ Providing alternative perspectives.
- ☑ Helping people get back on track after mistakes.
- ☑ Minimizing damage and speed recovery time after a mistake.
- ☑ Determining the cause of mistakes.
- ☑ Studying the elements of the perfect food plan in much more detail than could be accomplished in this book alone...
- ☑ Making each other's food plans better and better...
- ☑ Providing a constructive, cooperative, and loving atmosphere so everyone feels comfortable to take risks and grow...
- ☑ And much, much more!

In short, a community really does supercharge growth in the *Defeat Your Cravings* process, provided you can sidestep the notions of childlike *dependency* which can develop in unsupervised groups. Everyone must be supported to feel they *can* recover on their own, it's just that the group and coaching support supercharges the whole process. And it makes for a quicker, stronger, and more permanent recovery from cravings and overeating. *(Plus, now we've also added one-on-one coaching to the program, so you get the best of both worlds.)*

DO IT YOURSELF ADVICE

You can assemble your own group of individuals to accomplish these things independently if you wish. The idea is to find a crew willing to read, discuss, and implement the book together. You can often find such willing participants on social media groups that discuss overeating and food cravings, approach family and friends about the project, or even talk to people at your gym, yoga studio, or library *(if they offer self-help lectures where people are trying to improve themselves.)*

When organizing independent communities to study and implement the *Defeat Your Cravings* method, I recommend establishing a solid set of ground rules. Most notably, these should include most notably the idea of respecting people's autonomous food choices. Without this principle in place – *and someone assigned to police it* – the group may deteriorate into endless infighting about dietary philosophy. Which is better for you, ketogenic versus whole food plant based? Should you count calories, points, or carbs? Is fruit good or bad for you? How much protein do you need each day?

Even when you recruit experts, you'll find they rarely agree 100% of the time. People naturally want everyone to eat the way they're eating, because, well, as far as they're concerned it would just be a lot easier that way! Plus, the shorter amount of time people have followed their dietary style the more emphatic they are about it. It's almost as if before people feel solid enough to do it on their own, they want to eagerly convince everyone else to join them. Unfortunately, if you're not careful, the passion for this interferes with most constructive group activities. Okay, enough said about that.

The other critical ground rule when establishing independent groups is the idea of discouraging the perpetual dependency mindset. Accountability should be thought of as something temporary, like a cocoon built around new habits to protect you while you're developing them.

Our culture often encourages perpetual dependency when it comes to overcoming eating problems and other addictions. In fact, there are entire programs built on the notion of lifelong subjugation of your will to other people. When I was in such a program I was told, *"You've already proven yourself incapable of managing food on your own, Glenn. You need to report to a sponsor every day for the rest of your life. You had your chance, and you blew it. You'll need this level of accountability forever now."*

Nonsense!

What a disempowering message. *"You screwed up on your own so obviously you're incapable of doing otherwise. Your only hope is to become a dependent little child, forever looking to someone else to tell you what to eat."* How is that mindset really going to help anyone in the long run?

Perpetual accountability teaches your Pig that you're too weak to control it. As you know by now, there's a very well-established process for extinguishing your cravings. Using accountability as a tool to help you power through the extinction curves is a great idea. Moving in with your accountability partner so that they can keep an eye on you for the rest of your life is not!

To avoid that, you'll want to be sure the group is cultivating confidence and independence among members, not encouraging dependence. You'll know things are going in the wrong direction if people start saying, "We really need each other," or "I can't do it without you." An effective group leader fosters independence, and, ideally, interdependence, *not* dependence. The same goes for accountability buddies.

The last ground rule to establish when working with a group, is, ideally, maintaining attendance. Especially in small groups, if people have the tendency to hide after mistakes, having fewer individuals attend the meeting really lowers the energy and potential value of the group. This impact is less severe in larger groups, but it's still a good idea to encourage people to show up no matter what, and to make sure nobody is belittled or demeaned for their mistakes. The group leader needs to be on the alert, so this kind of criticism is redirected, and participants always feel safe and supported.

Putting together an effective, independent support group to study and implement *Defeat Your Cravings* method. I can also be a difficult task because different people have varying levels of motivation at different times in their lives, and not everyone takes to the concept. That being said, it can be difficult for an individual to find enough people with the right level of motivation and interest to keep the program moving effectively. Plus, implementing the above ground rules is not easy.

That's why I've developed two levels of *Defeat Your Cravings* community support. *(Available as of the date of publication.)*

01. **Our free readers community** allows you to connect with other readers, listen to hundreds of demonstration sessions and interviews about the *Defeat Your Cravings* process *(and its predecessor.)* Get into the free community and download the free smartphone app at www.DefeatYourCravings.com

02. **Our online accountability, group support, and individual coaching program** is an extremely powerful, three-month program where your individual accountability coach will walk you through the *Defeat Your Cravings* process step by step.

There's a group call every day of the week including weekends, so you're never more than 24 hours away from talking to an experienced coach directly. At present, I run the group calls myself four days per week while my highly trained and experienced coaches run the group sessions the rest of the days each week. I can't promise to do this forever though, so if this interests you, it's best to join now.

Educational videos are also available for each of the steps in this book. They'll always include the most up-to-date information as well as tips and tricks, and many bonus webinars, cheat sheets, and workshops. Plus, you'll get an unlimited number of individual sessions with your one-on-one coach, provided you work on the process in between sessions. Yes, you read that right. Unlimited. See the details on the site please.

Of course, I can't provide this level of support for free as I must train, pay, and supervise my coaches, and there's a significant amount of my personal time involved, but I think you'll find it very affordable for everything you get. Details are on the site at www.DefeatYourCravingsCoaching.com

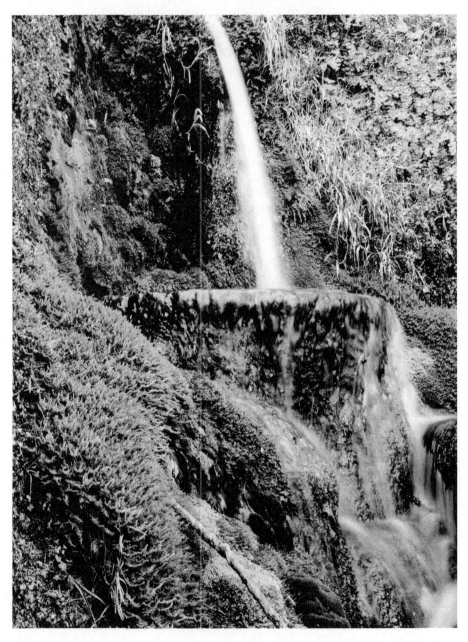

FROM THE BOTTOM OF MY HEART TO THE BOTTOM OF YOURS

I know you can do this. I really do! I believe my decades of suffering were not in vein but serve a greater purpose. I'm not entirely sure what I believe about God or why I was put on this planet, but I do know that helping people defeat their cravings is about the most meaningful, fulfilling work I've ever done. Witnessing people overcome their deep pain *(as I personally experienced at the mercy of my Pig)—and witnessing the liberation they feel when they realize they can defeat it*—fills me with awe and appreciation.

So, from the bottom of my heart to the bottom of yours, thank you for your time, attention, and willingness to even consider this solution. My only hope is that you will implement it even a little and experience even one-tenth of the freedom it has given me.

All my love,

Glenn
P.S. *"A man who is a slave to his impulses is surely not free."* – Seneca

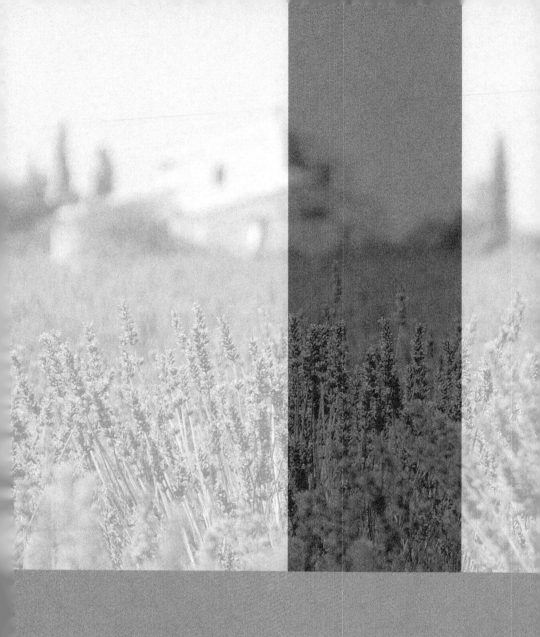

APPENDIX

Appendix A
HOW TO REFUTE THE MOST COMMON SQUEALS

ONE BITE WON'T HURT

"One bite won't hurt," "Just a little will be fine," "Just eat it; it won't hurt this one time," "This time it'll really only be one bite," "Just once, you'll feel so much better," "It's just a little bit; nobody's perfect after all," "Just this once won't matter."

Odds are you've heard these words more than once in your life, and, like most clients, have given in to them more than once too. The good news is, there are many strong ways to disempower them.

First, most people's Pigs Squeal call out for some industrially created, highly concentrated food, specifically designed to stimulate cravings – substances that hyper-energize your lizard brain with stimulants like sugar, caffeine, and theobromine – flavors like spicy, salty, sweet, or sour – and condensed sources of energy like sugar, fats, oils, carbs, etc. We didn't have these things on the savannah, so they "light up" the "find calories" mechanism in the brain like a bonfire in a paper store, quickly creating addictive pathways likely to be repeated. One bite can be the difference between strengthening these pathways versus weakening them. Also, by energizing your lizard brain, these foods dampen your higher cognitive functions – *rational decision making, focus on long term goals, etc.* – making it harder to resist the *next* bite.

Then there's the fact that "just one bite" almost always conceals a secondary, more dangerous Squeal. See, after taking one bite off your food plan, your Pig will probably deliver a second punch. *"Screw it, you already blew it!"* it will say. After this one-two punch, it will push for you to eat whatever you want for the rest of the day, leading to a big giant binge, ruined weight loss, disturbed sleep, and abject misery. So, what the Pig *really* means by *"One bite won't hurt,"* is *"One big giant binge won't hurt!"* But it's not stupid, it knows you'd see right through this if it were honest, so it breaks the Squeal into two parts to soften you up first.

Third, even though as a practical matter most people make at least some mistakes along the way, *repeatedly* taking one bite off your food plan might cause you to lose faith in the process entirely. It's the difference between being the master of your destiny with food versus a constant slave to your cravings and impulses. Do this often enough and you'll develop feelings of hopelessness, helplessness, and powerlessness, which can lead to months *(or even years)* of letting your cravings run the show and all the misery that entails.

Fourth, when you reward the Pig for squealing, the Squeals get stronger. That's how the brain works. But interfering with the urge-reward loop dramatically decreases both cravings and food obsession over time. The brain is very efficient and sees no use in continuing to generate strong cravings and excuses to indulge them when these impulses are no longer rewarded.

Fifth, breaking promises to yourself downgrades your self-esteem. Your Pig knows this and will use it to make you feel too weak to resist the next binge. Remember, the Pig is sociopathic by definition and only cares about Slop, not how much it hurts you in the process.

Sixth, consistency matters. One bite is the difference between consistently being on plan versus off plan, and between consistently moving toward your goals versus moving away from your goals. What you habitually do in the face of temptation defines your character. Embracing consistent eating within your food rules builds confidence and eradicates the constant thinking about food. Eventually your Pig will learn there's no point in throwing its crazy ideas at you because they never work, and your mind will be free to think about more important things.

Seventh, every craving is an opportunity for self-love versus self-harm. Love yourself by seizing the opportunity to re-train yourself to crave healthy things instead. For example, I overcame my chocolate addiction by having green smoothies when the cravings hit. Eventually I craved smoothies, not chocolate. In contrast, indulging a craving reinforces destructive patterns *(self-harm)*. Breaking your rules is a way of telling yourself, *"You and your dreams do not matter."*

Eighth, if you eat some junk now, you'll still need to eat something healthy later. Your body screams for a certain amount of nourishment each day no matter what. Since "just one bite" of empty calories usually adds up to 1,000 to 3,000 after the "screw it, you already blew it" Squeal that follows, you'll wind up with *extra* calories for the day, often enough to gain a half pound or more.

Ninth, you wouldn't tell an ex-smoker, "Just one cigarette won't hurt," would you? You previously decided to commit to a food rule at a time when you were of sound mind and body and had the fortitude to recognize there was an addictive pattern developing. You decided this pattern was interfering with your life and that you wanted to defeat it. This was a sacred commitment. If it helps, think of "one bite off your plan" as being equally as dangerous as telling an ex-smoker "just one cigarette."

Tenth, would you say yes to a vampire who said, "C'mon, just one bite!" Expose your neck to a vampire and it will suck *all* your blood. The Pig is no different, so don't offer it "just one bite" of your neck!

One bite off your plan *does* hurt. In fact, one bite off plan is a tragedy.

YOU NEED COMFORT FOOD – YOU'RE TOO UPSET TO EAT HEALTHILY

The idea you "need" to overeat to deal with your emotions is one of the most common misconceptions in the modern world. Alternative forms of this lie include specific emotions to fear: anger, loneliness, excitement, sadness, rebelliousness, and anxiety.

If you eat for emotional reasons, you should know the relationship between overeating and emotional upset is much more complex than you realize. Most people think they overindulge their cravings out of a need for comfort and escape from difficult and unpleasant emotions. This is a broad generalization which both exaggerates the reality and fails to acknowledge several other very important factors involved.

The nervous system has difficulty conducting its emotions when the digestive system is overloaded, so overeating does have an anesthetic effect. That's why people who think of "comfort food" believe they're indulging to escape or "numb out." But if your dentist were out of Novocain, would she offer to inject you with a bagel instead? No! So, there must be something else going on here.

In addition to "numbing out" and escaping, you're doing something else when you indulge. You are "getting high with food." People tend to indulge in artificial concentrations of pleasure that don't exist in nature. It might be perfectly legal, but another name for such things is a drug. Changing your paradigm from "I'm eating for comfort," to "My Pig wants to get high with food," will help you tremendously. Only apply this to foods and behaviors that break your rules.

Next, the desire to escape an unpleasant emotion may create an urge to overeat, but the urge must first be justified before becoming behavior. The reason is, when you commit to a particular way of behaving and observe yourself about to break this commitment, you experience what Leon Festinger called "cognitive dissonance," a psychologically uncomfortable state (Festinger 1957).

In plain English, people prefer to think of themselves as having a consistent and reliable character, and every food rule is a kind of character commitment. *"I will never again eat chocolate on a weekday,"* really means, *"I've chosen to become the kind of person who only eats chocolate on weekends."* Eating chocolate on a Wednesday doesn't jibe with this commitment, so your brain will try to rationalize it. "It's okay because I worked out hard enough, so it doesn't matter," or "I deserve a treat once in a while; it's been a very hard day," etc. Refutations prevent rationalization and can make it too uncomfortable to allow yourself to break the rule.

Finally, most people are very surprised to know that the emotion-overeating relationship is bidirectional. It goes both ways. As described in Step Six, there's a very well-established psychological principle called operant conditioning: A behavior and/or thought followed by a reward will be more likely to recur *(recall my dog learning to sneeze for cheese)*.

It's not just behavior that can be operantly conditioned though, emotional states can, too, when they're followed by a food reward. They become more likely to be amplified and repeated. For example, many people say they must overeat before bed, or they'll feel too anxious to sleep. I explain that anxiety has a lot of physical correlates such as higher respiration, heart rate, blood pressure, galvanic skin response, pupillary dilation, etc. I tell them animal studies on groups of orangutans, for example, show they can be conditioned to have consistently higher blood pressure when given a sugar reward whenever their pressure goes up.

So, it may be that overeating is creating anxiety not the other way around. Or it may be the relationship is bidirectional. Anxiety stimulates overeating, and overeating stimulates anxiety. Either way, you can often break the cycle by not overeating in response to anxiety no matter what. I've had many clients who've done this tell me that within a few weeks they're miraculously able to sleep without Slop. Not all of them, but most.

This same process is at play for other emotions too. Your Pig may say sugar is the only relief from depression you can find, but what if sugar is the reason for depression in the first place? What if eating sugar every time you feel depressed is making you *more* depressed?

Food for thought!

Also, your emotional issues may have been the match that started the fire, but once it started burning, that fire probably took on a life of its own. Once a craving is programmed into your personal neurology, deprogramming it requires practical methods discussed in this book, not deep psychological insights.

Because of this complex relationship between overeating and emotion, emotional insight alone usually will not stop you from overeating. It may improve your life independently of your eating, but it's not the primary route I suggest you take in your quest to defeat your cravings. As long as you think you must overcome all your emotional issues to stop overeating, or believe you're only eating for "comfort," you'll just be giving your Pig one more excuse to keep indulging.

There are a few practical takeaways. First, don't tell yourself you're overeating for emotional reasons, to relieve stress, to "cope," or to comfort yourself. That's a mindset which feeds the fire and gives your Pig an excuse: *"You're WAY too upset. These feelings are awful. You simply must go get comfort food to escape them!"* Tell yourself you overeat to get high with food, much like a drug addict might do with drugs. This will make it more uncomfortable to keep doing it.

Then, decide you're willing to go through *any* level of emotional discomfort to stick to your rule. This way you won't continue to distract yourself or waste valuable energy on recovering from overeating in addition to the emotional struggle. Energy becomes more available to *solve* problems. *"The only way out is through!"*

My grandfather used to say, *"If you've got six problems and choose to overeat, you'll then have seven problems."* For example, suppose you're stressed about money and decide to indulge some off-plan cravings as a distraction. You'll get a maximum of one hour of relief while the high from the Slop lasts, and thereafter you'll still be financially stressed. The only difference is, now you'll also feel bloated and self-conscious from all the Slop passing through your body. You'll probably also sleep badly and wake up cranky. So, you were stressed out about money, but now you're *also* feeling ashamed, guilty, bloated, and tired. That's not what you wanted to achieve, is it?

But if you resist the craving and stay on plan, you'll feel more confident, in control, and have more energy. I'm not saying the money problems will go away overnight – *and by the way I was approximately $700,000 in debt in 2003, so I'm not talking just talking theory* – but these mental resources will be available to help you to cope and work on the financial issues. Now, that's better!

> **Let your Pig know you're willing to feel any degree of emotional discomfort to not break your food rules.**

I distinctly remember having to implement these insights about emotional eating the week my Mom got diagnosed with the final recurrence of ovarian cancer, which would take her life three months later, right around the same time I was going through a breakup.

Unfortunately, life isn't a pain-free experience. Happiness is not guaranteed just because you stop overeating. What you get when you eliminate overeating is *your life* – for better or for worse. Marry your life, not your Pig. It's much better to be present no matter the pain than to spend days, weeks, or months recovering from overeating. Overeating is a waste of life, no matter how painful that life may become.

Once you *really* understand this, you'll stop letting emotions confuse the issue. Oh, you'll still have them, perhaps even more so, but you'll understand they don't run the show. It took me decades to get this, and I'll never get those years back, so I'd like to save you the pain!

Lastly, please don't let anything above stop you from consulting a licensed physician and following their advice. There is a real role for medication, psychotherapy, and professional treatment in overcoming emotional struggles, and some truly are biochemical in origin. I'm just saying the above factors are also in play, and the Pig's simplistic explanation that you "need" the Slop for comfort to escape from the negative feelings is bogus.

YOU MUST FIND THE PERFECT DIET FIRST

Often the Pig will Squeal that you first must research and decide upon the perfect diet before committing to even one simple rule. Usually when a person lives with this kind of Squeal, they've tried diet after diet, jumping from one to the next, never giving any of them enough time to see if they will work. This destroys their confidence because these individuals come to believe they can't stick to anything, and that nothing will ever work.

Alternatively, I call this the "Confuse and Conquer" Squeal because that's the Pig's goal – to keep the debate going forever so it can live in the resulting rule vacuum. See, there'll *always* be controversy about which dietary philosophy is best, so requiring a perfect understanding of the most optimal diet for humans before changing behavior is a losing game.

The only way to beat this lie is to remember it's better to stay on *any* reasonable plan for a few months than to jump from plan to plan. This is true even if the plan you're working with is flawed. It's better to have at least *some* rules in place than to allow chaos to reign, because in the absence of rules, your Pig will have a field day. Giving your intellect control over your emotions and whims where difficult food decisions are concerned requires committing to at least one crystal-clear food rule.

> **The grass is not greener on the other side; the grass is greener where it's watered.**

Another way to beat this lie is to require a minimum of seven days before any written changes to your food rules take effect. This way you can't ever change your plan impulsively based upon the Pig's whims and whines.

JUST START AGAIN TOMORROW

I've already talked about the final two common Pig Squeals when illustrating refutation, but because they are so common and *so* powerful, I will more thoroughly eradicate the cancerous logic here.

> **"Let's overeat today, it'll be just as easy to start your silly diet again tomorrow" is the most common lie which causes people to think permanently defeating their cravings is impossible.**

Variations include: *"One last time," "Today doesn't count because [insert reason here] – you can just start again in the morning," "You're getting good at getting back on track before too much damage is done, so go ahead and binge today, it won't be so bad and you can get on the plan for real tomorrow,"* etc.

There are seven reasons this line of reasoning is clearly false. By studying them you can thoroughly disempower this awful belief before it ruins your confidence.

First, scientific studies demonstrate that if you indulge today, it will be harder to ignore cravings tomorrow. On the other hand, if you stay on plan today it will be *easier* to eat healthy tomorrow. Research into the neuroplasticity of learning shows we are always either reinforcing or extinguishing our food patterns, so there is really no standing still. It won't be "just as easy" to begin again tomorrow, it will be harder. If you're in a hole, stop digging!

Second, you can't eat tomorrow, you can only eat *now*, because when tomorrow comes, it will be *now* again! The purpose of the "start tomorrow" Squeal is to deny this fundamental fact and focus on the future instead of the present moment. The Pig wants to make overeating seem okay *now*. When you realize the only time you can put food in your mouth is the present moment, and that it's always the present (*e.g., when tomorrow comes it will be the present again*), then you'll know how to push this silly thought out of your head.

If you never indulge *now*, you'll never indulge *again* because the future is an infinite string of present moments. During absolutely every second it took you to read this paragraph it was the present moment, and as a matter of fact, it still is! So, when the "let's start tomorrow" idea pops into your head just say to yourself, *"I always use the present moment to be healthy,"* or *"I never overeat now,"* and you'll be fine.

Third, the more you flex your "eat healthy now" muscle the stronger it gets, so the Pig's prediction that it will be easier to "get you later" when you're not so vigilant is false as well. The more you use the present moment to eat healthy, the harder it becomes for the Pig to get you, especially since cravings die down over time if you don't reward them.

Fourth, every bite counts, every last one! Your brain may be able to wrap itself around the false notion that what you eat today doesn't count because you'll make up for it "tomorrow" *(which never comes),* but your body can't. Each and every bite you take either nourishes you or saps your health. Every wrong decision reinforces the addiction and every right one weakens it. Every bite counts, no matter what no matter what no matter what!

Fifth, your word is sacred. Knowing you can keep a promise to yourself means everything. Being able to stick to a plan is the foundation of self-mastery, which is what allows you to accomplish virtually everything else in life. For this reason, "one bite" off your food rules *today* can ruin your belief in yourself tomorrow and interfere with the rest of your life in more profound ways than you realize. You need to know you'll do what you say you're going to do – it's exceptionally important.

Sixth, if you give the Pig even one inch off your carefully defined food plan you know it will take a mile! That's why one bite off your diet is too many, even though your Pig will say 1,000 bites are not enough. *(I didn't make that up.)* Tomorrow never comes. Always use the present moment to be healthy.

Seventh, the Pig may beg for "one last time," but you know when you do that, there's always one more, right? How many "last suppers" are you going to feed it?

YOU'VE FAILED 1,000 TIMES BEFORE

The *"You've failed 1,000 times before so you must fail again,"* Squeal comes in several alternate forms. You may have heard: *"You'll just gain all the weight back again (and more)," "You know you'll break your stupid diet eventually, so why not give up now and be happy with that already!"; "You've been doing this for X years and have spent Y dollars trying Z diet programs, so why on earth will this be any different?"; "You've proven you can't do this a thousand times already, why bother again?"*

The idea that you've always failed in the past so you must always fail in the future fools most people into believing permanent progress is impossible, but it's an easy idea to beat when you know how!

First, recognize that the negative self-talk about mistakes is the Pig's activity, motivated only by the desire to eat more Slop! The Pig's whole purpose in beating you down about your past failures is to make you feel too weak to resist overeating *today*. It turns out to be very difficult to keep overeating if you refuse to keep criticizing yourself.

Second, remind yourself that continuing to get up and try again is a sign of strength, not weakness! Your Pig thinks it's putting you down with this idea when it's actually complimenting you! How many of the world's most significant accomplishments were made by people who got it right on the first try? Even if you've repeatedly fallen down for years, continuing to get up until you succeed is a mark of strength, not weakness!

People who keep getting up and trying are much more likely to eventually find a way to lose weight and keep it off. I mean, duh!

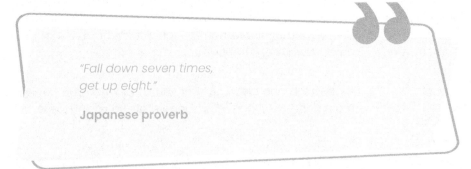

*"Fall down seven times,
get up eight."*

Japanese proverb

Furthermore, research suggests one of the primary distinctions between long-term weight loss and yo-yo dieting is the sheer number of attempts.

Permanent weight loss is more often achieved by people with more failures behind them. The name of the game clearly is staying in the game until you win the game!

Third, train yourself to collect evidence of success, not of failure. See, you can choose which lens to use to gather evidence about your life and experiences. In fact, perhaps the biggest choice you'll ever make is whether to utilize the lens of success versus the lens of failure. Your Pig wants you to choose the lens of failure so you can build a failure identity and keep indulging your cravings. Choose the lens of success to build a success mindset instead. **Make a habit of writing down what you did right each week with food, no matter what you did wrong!**

Fourth, as I've said before, remember that even if you've driven on a highway for a thousand miles without taking an exit, you can still take the next one! There is *nothing* which compels you to stay on a highway that's taking you in the wrong direction. To the best of my knowledge there is no law that states you aren't allowed to turn around or to turn the wheel at all.

THIS IS TOO HARD! YOU'LL BE TORTURED WITH CRAVINGS FOREVER!

There are several reasons why the idea that disciplining yourself with a set of food rules will feel indefinitely torturous is false. First, people who successfully keep weight off after losing it tend to develop intrinsic motivation which turns them into a different kind of person with regard to food. Successful weight loss people don't see themselves as dieters anymore. Instead, they enjoy the process and the journey of changing their eating identity.

They also tend to switch their motivation as they near their goal weight. Cravings die down dramatically as a result of eating on plan for so long. The Pig learns there's no point in continuing to pester them to break rules when these efforts are never rewarded. It becomes less about weight loss and more about enjoying their new lifestyle, free from yo-yo dieting and food obsession.

They recall their previous obsession with food and cravings as torture but feel this is finally behind them.

So, the initial answer is that disciplined eating is only torturous when you choose to *make* it torturous. You don't have to do that. You can choose a very comfortable plan provided your doctor says there's no emergency to lose weight fast.

But there are two more answers to the "discipline is way too hard" lie. The first has to do with the neurological principles of downregulation and upregulation discussed previously. Your cravings will *not* last forever, even though your Pig says you'll be tortured indefinitely by them. Your nervous system will become more responsive to natural pleasures once you stop overstimulating it with unnatural ones. So, the Pig says you'll be tortured forever without its favorite Slop, but it's lying! When I stopped eating chocolate to lose weight, I stopped having cravings after only a few months. The very same thing happened to me with flour. It took about eight weeks for 80% of the cravings to go away. Around the six months mark they were only 5% of what they once were.

Unfortunately, this extinction curve gets reset every time you indulge. It turns out we're almost always downregulating or upregulating, there's really no in-between. So, if cravings are bothering you, the best thing to do is *stay* on your plan so it will get easier – the exact opposite of what your Pig is arguing for!

Also, remember you'll be depriving yourself more by continuing to indulge than by changing your habits, due to the two types of deprivation previously discussed. The negative impacts of continuing to indulge last forever, but the feelings of deprivation while extinguishing cravings are only temporary – it's much, much more painful to continue giving in!

Finally, who says there's got to be an "easy" way? Many key paths in life require choosing between two difficult alternatives.

Alternative forms of the "you'll be too deprived" Squeal include the following: *"You simply can't give up that much pleasure"; "Food is your only real pleasure and you'll suffer too much without unlimited access to whatever you want"; "I'll make your life unbearable forever by constantly asking for more."*

Appendix B
WHAT IF IT DOESN'T WORK?

01. **Medical problems may underlie certain cravings that don't succumb to these techniques.** See a licensed physician to rule these out.

02. **I've witnessed miracles in people who seemingly couldn't "get it" for years when they finally adopted a food plan with no sugar, flour, or alcohol.** With the permission of a licensed physician, consider adopting the following three very specific rules for 90 days: (a) The only sweet taste I will ever eat again is whole fruit; (b) The only starches I will ever eat again are potatoes and whole grains; (c) I will never again drink alcohol.

Extra credit if you can add a full pound of un-sauced leafy green vegetables every day, assuming there is no reason this is medically contraindicated. (*You can even put them in a blender with some water and drink them down, you don't have to go through the hassle of making a big salad.*)

Remember: You can adjust these with conditional rules after the 90 days are up, but the idea is to be very strict until then. No artificial sweeteners, no special flour exceptions, and zero alcohol. No playing around. And no under-eating! Being sure you get enough calories and nutrition is even more important if you're undertaking this plan. Lose weight slowly.

03. **Eliminate as much stimulation as possible for 30 days.** *Defeat Your Cravings* is a take-no-prisoners, aggressive approach to overcoming overeating. The idea is to seize the day and cultivate confidence rather than fear! I want you to be able to spontaneously go to your favorite restaurant with your friends and stare down the most tempting dishes without breaking your rules. I joke with people, but it's true, that you could fill up my bathtub with chocolate and force me to bathe in it and I still wouldn't eat any.

That said, sometimes protecting yourself from stimulation is very helpful, particularly if you'll be giving up some serious binging on sugar, flour, salt, and alcohol, and particularly for the first ten days. It's everywhere. So, take a different route home from work to avoid passing that bakery. Ask the kids to keep their chips and ice cream someplace you can't see it, or even in a separate cabinet or freezer. Avoid watching commercials on television for a while. Don't go out to eat for ten days. The idea is to create a cocoon around your new habits so you can get beyond the tantrum phase of the extinction burst *(please see the chapter on extinguishing your cravings if you don't know what that means.)*

Then, as you're feeling more confident, you can slowly expose yourself to the stimulation again. Watch out for the trap of cultivating permanent isolation from stimulation or becoming frightened of the world. You can't avoid food signals, they're everywhere, and if the only way you can control your cravings is to isolate yourself from the world, you'll be retreating to a very small world indeed. In my previous program, for example, we ran into people who had their kids lock them in their room so they couldn't raid the refrigerator at night. This is not a practical way to live your life!

The idea is to gradually deal with increasingly more *(and more intense)* food signals until you feel like there's nothing you can't do. I never actually had anyone fill a bathtub with chocolate and throw me in it. But after I was free of chocolate cravings for about 90 days, I *did* go to the supermarket several times and stood right in front of my previous nemesis in the chocolate aisle. I did this on days I was well nourished and had already asked my Pig what its best reason for indulging today might be – I brought along a preemptive refutation just in case. Then I went in and stood there and said *"Go ahead, Mr. Pig, give me one good reason to buy this and eat it."* The Pig had nothing. *Nothing!* It was very empowering.

As with everything else in the *Defeat Your Cravings* method, you don't want to jump right into this type of thought experiment. Start small and work your way up. For example, I went to a birthday party where I knew there would be chocolate party favors but plenty of other people around. *(I never binged in front of others, so this wasn't a big risk for me.)* Then, I also went out for coffee with a friend who bought brownies at Starbucks. I acclimated to the chocolate stimulation gradually and maintained my confidence throughout.

04. Get enough rest. I touched on this briefly in the chapter on turning off false alarms, but, after a paucity of nutrition and calories *(over-restriction)*, lack of rest is probably the worst culprit for creating "irresistible" cravings. Rest replenishes willpower and the ability to make good decisions. There's really no substitute. Just rest up.

05. Manage "that time of the month." Research suggests overeating and body dissatisfaction are elevated when progesterone levels rise during the premenstrual phase of your cycle. Moreover, appetite rises when estrogen levels are lowest, which happens to be during your cycle *(highest during ovulation).* Leading up to and for the duration of your period you are physiologically predisposed to be unhappy with yourself and will want to devour food!

On the other hand, your metabolism may be slightly elevated during the luteal phase just before your period due to increased thyroid function. All things considered, it can be helpful to create a conditional rule which allows 5% to 10% extra nutrition and calories *(not junk)* during this time of the month. Magnesium-rich foods such as spinach, avocados, and/or black beans, as well as foods rich in B6 vitamins such as carrots, peas, bananas, and chickpeas can be particularly helpful because they may boost your serotonin levels and lessen the severity of cravings. Eating 30g to 35g of non-fruit carbohydrates *(e.g., quinoa and other whole grains)* may similarly boost serotonin levels. As always, check with your doctor before changing your diet.

See Racine et al. (2011) and Wurtman (2010) for more information on hormonal shifts and preventing PMS from wreaking havoc on your food plan.

06. Beat the "grass is greener on the other side" syndrome: Do you ever feel confused about which diet to follow? One day it's keto, the next one of those calorie-counting or points systems? If you could just stop jumping from diet to diet you might be fine, but you don't know which

one to choose because they all seem right *and* they all seem wrong? This is the result of the Pig's attempts to confuse and conquer with something called "The Grass is Greener on the Other Side" syndrome.

You see, in a state of uncertainty, the Pig wins. If there are no clear rules then, the Pig reasons, anything goes. That's why it wants you to be constantly confused about what diet and/or food plan to follow, and why it "trash talks" about various dietary philosophies in the same way boxers psych out their opponents. Most great boxers use TV interviews, social media, and every opportunity they can find to convince would-be opponents that they're too weak to step in the ring with them. "I'll break you, leave you bloodied and humiliated on the boxing-ring floor for your family and friends to see, you worthless, stupid loser. You don't stand a chance!"

The trash talk continues all the way up to the fight... even inside the ring they continue trash talking with the goal of making their opponent forget their plan. And that's how they can calmly step up to that poor other guy and knock him out.

The Pig is doing the very same thing to get *you* to jump from diet to diet. *"Hey, you've tried this diet for a whole week (or month, etc.) and you haven't lost any weight! In fact, you actually gained a little, and you had to cheat a bunch because this is obviously not the right diet for you... so just go on to the next one. In the meantime, you can eat tons of Slop, right? Pretty please!!?"* – Your Pig

The solution is picking *one* plan that's anywhere close to reasonable and sticking to it, even if it's not perfect. People do much better when they have a clear target to aim for. It's just too tempting to eat anything and everything when you don't. If the dietary philosophy you're following turns out to be less than perfect, you can modify it later. Consult a dietitian, doctor, or nutritionist for help. Just don't allow a state of uncertainty to prevail because that is a losing game.

"The grass isn't greener on the other side, the grass is greener where it's watered" - Robert Fulghum.

07. Stop trying to convince other people to eat like you do. Unless and until you've truly defeated your cravings for six months and are feeling very confident and strong, stay out of debates and discussions about the right way to eat. It only aggravates other people's Pigs, who will then throw their

worst Squeals at you because they don't want to give up their Slop. You've got enough to manage with your own Pig, don't engage others.

08. Dealing with Nighttime Overeating: Eat a more substantial breakfast, and a significant lunch, which includes some crunchy vegetables or crunchy fruit. Don't save the bulk of your calories for nighttime. The vast majority of nighttime overeaters who overcame this problem in our programs were unconsciously saving calories for later in the day. Eat breakfast and add crunch to your lunch!

You can also stair-step your way to a 100% no nighttime overeating rule instead of trying to get there right away. For example, instead of saying, *"I'll never again eat anything after 8 p.m.,"* you can say, *"I'll never again eat anything besides un-sauced vegetables, tea, and almond milk after 8 p.m."* Or allow yourself a 100-calorie healthy snack. Something with a clear boundary.

Appendix C
DRUGS AND ALCOHOL

Do you struggle with drugs, alcohol, or other black-and-white addictions? If so, I recommend Jack Trimpey's *Rational Recovery* book over anything I've ever written. Don't try to define an "Alcohol Pig" or "Drug Pig" and apply the *Defeat Your Cravings* methodology; instead, use his methods, which you'll find compatible with the philosophy in this book.

There is some significant overlap, in fact, because reading Mr. Trimpey's books were the first to introduce me to the idea of clearly separating constructive from destructive thoughts in addiction, as well as the idea that addiction is not a disease but a choice and misapplication of free will and responsibility – there are also some very clear distinctions. These distinctions are of sufficient magnitude that drug and alcohol addictions will *not* succumb to my methods as outlined in this book in the same way that food will.

I've also never seriously struggled with drugs, alcohol, or cigarettes on a personal level, so I don't feel I'm the best representative to help people overcome these addictions. *(I really hate never-addicted professionals who stand up and say they really understand!)* Moreover, I haven't studied drug and alcohol addiction in the same comprehensive manner I've studied food.

For these reasons, you're much better off reading Mr. Trimpey's body of work if these particular substances have you caught in the Venus Fly Trap of toxic pleasure. You can still find his books on Amazon.com as of the date of this publication.

Appendix D
REFERENCES

01. Blum, K., Thanos, P. K., & Gold, M. S. (2014). Dopamine and glucose, obesity, and reward deficiency syndrome. *Frontiers in Psychology, 5.* https://doi.org/10.3389/fpsyg.2014.00919

02. Center for Disease Control and Prevention (2023, January 5). *Obesity and Overweight.* Retrieved May 31, 2023, from https://www.cdc.gov/nchs/fastats/obesity-overweight.htm

03. Chao, A., Loughead, J., Bakizada, Z., Hopkins, C., Geliebter, A., Gur, R., & Wadden, T. (2017). Sex/gender differences in neural correlates of food stimuli: a systematic review of functional neuroimaging studies. Obesity Reviews.

04. Donaldson, M. S., Nutrition and cancer: a review of the evidence for an anti-cancer diet. Journal of Nutrition. 2004 Oct 20;3:19. doi: 10.1186/1475-2891-3-19. PMID: 15496224; PMCID: PMC526387.

05. Festinger, L. (1957). *A Theory of Cognitive Dissonance.* Stanford University Press. https://www.amazon.com/Theory-Cognitive-Dissonance-Leon-Festinger/dp/0804709114/

06. Grenon, R., Schwartze, D., Hammond, N., Ivanova, I., Mcquaid, N., Proulx, G., & Tasca, G. (2017). Group psychotherapy for eating disorders: A meta⊠ analysis. International Journal of Eating Disorders.

07. Harvard T.H. Chan School of Public Health (n.d.). *Simple Steps to Preventing Diabetes*. Harvard.edu. Retrieved May 31, 2023, from https://www.hsph.harvard.edu/nutritionsource/disease-prevention/diabetes-prevention/preventing-diabetes-full-story/

08. Juhaeri, J., Stevens, J., Chambless, L., Tyroler, H., Harp, J., Jones, D., & Arnett, D. (2004). Weight change among self-reported dieters and non-dieters in white and African American men and women. European Journal of Epidemiology. https://doi.org/10.1023/A:1016270128624.

09. Kawa, A. B., Allain, F., Robinson, T. E., & Samaha, A.-N. (2019). The transition to cocaine addiction: The importance of pharmacokinetics for preclinical models. *Psychopharmacology*, *236*(4), 1145–1157. https://doi.org/10.1007/s00213-019-5164-0

10. Kenny, P. J., Voren, G., & Johnson, P. M. (2013). Dopamine D2 receptors and striatopallidal transmission in addiction and obesity. *Current Opinion in Neurobiology*, *23*(4), 535–538. https://doi.org/10.1016/j.conb.2013.04.012

11. Latner, J., & Ciao, A. (2014). Weight-loss history as a predictor of obesity treatment outcome: Prospective, long-term results from behavioral, group self-help treatment. Journal of Health Psychology.

12. Mantantzis K., Schlaghecken F., Sünram-Lea, S.I., Maylor, E.A. Sugar rush or sugar crash? A meta-analysis of carbohydrate effects on mood. Neuroscience Biobehavioral Rev. 2019 Jun;101:45-67. doi: 10.1016/j.neubiorev.2019.03.016. Epub 2019 Apr 3. PMID: 30951762.

13. Market Data Forecast (2023, March 1). *Global Fresh Fruits and Vegetables Market Segmented By Product Type (Vegetables and Fruits), By End-Users (Inorganic and Organic), By Application (Commercial and Household), and Regional (North America, Europe, Asia Pacific, Latin America, and Middle East and Africa) – Global Industry Size, Share, Growth, Trends and Competitive Strategy Analysis Forecast (2023-2028)*. Retrieved June 25, 2023, from https://www.marketdataforecast.com/market-reports/fresh-fruits-and-vegetables-market

14. Miller, W., Franklin, B., Janosz, K., Vial, C., Kaitner, R., & McCullough, P. (2009). Advantages of group treatment and structured exercise in promoting short-term weight loss and cardiovascular risk reduction in adults with central obesity. Metabolic syndrome and related disorders.

15. Nakata, Y., Okada, M., Hashimoto, K., Harada, Y., Sone, H., & Tanaka, K. (2011). Comparison of Education-Only versus Group-Based Intervention in Promoting Weight Loss: A Randomised Controlled Trial. Obesity Facts.

16. Neumark⬛Sztainer, D., Wall, M., Haines, J., Story, M., & Eisenberg, M. (2007). Why does dieting predict weight gain in adolescents? Findings from project EAT-II: a five-year longitudinal study. Journal of the American Dietetic Association. https://doi.org/10.1016/J.JADA.2006.12.013.

17. Paakki, M., Sandell, M., & Hopia, A. (2019). Visual attractiveness depends on colorfulness and color contrasts in mixed salads. Food Quality and Preference.

18. Racine, S.E., Culbert, K.M., Keel, P.K., Sisk, C.L., Burt, S.A, Klump, K.L. (2011). Differential associations between ovarian hormones and disordered eating symptoms across the menstrual cycle in women. International Journal of Eating Disorders *(Vol 45, Issue 3, 333-334)*

19. Renjilian, D., Perri, M., Nezu, A., McKelvey, W., Shermer, R., & Anton, S. (2001). Individual versus group therapy for obesity: effects of matching participants to their treatment preferences. Journal of Consulting and Clinical Psychology.

20. Roitman, M., Stuber, G., Phillips, P., Wightman, R., & Carelli, R. (2004). Dopamine Operates as a Subsecond Modulator of Food Seeking. The Journal of Neuroscience.

21. Salamone, J. D., & Correa, M. (2013). Dopamine and Food Addiction: Lexicon Badly Needed. Biological Psychiatry, 73(9), e15–e24. https://doi.org/10.1016/j.biopsych.2012.09.027

22. Schultz, W. Dopamine signals for reward value and risk: basic and recent data. Behav Brain Funct 6, 24 (2010). https://doi.org/10.1186/1744-9081-6-24

23. Seligman, M. E. P. (2006). Learned Optimism: How To Change Your Mind And Your Life. Vintage Books.

24. Siahpush, M., Tibbits, M., Shaikh, R., Singh, G., Kessler, A., & Huang, T. (2015). Dieting Increases the Likelihood of Subsequent Obesity and BMI Gain: Results from a Prospective Study of an Australian National Sample. International Journal of Behavioral Medicine. https://doi.org/10.1007/s12529-015-9463-5.

25. Song, Z., Reinhardt, K., Buzdon, M., & Liao, P. (2008). Association between support group attendance and weight loss after Roux-en-Y gastric bypass. Surgery for obesity and related diseases: official journal of the American Society for Bariatric Surgery.

26. Singh, S. (2006), "Impact of color on marketing," Management Decision, Vol. 44, No. 6, pp. 783-789. https://doi.org/10.1108/00251740610673332.

27. Trief, P., Delahanty, L., Cibula, D., & Weinstock, R. (2018). Behavior Change of Participants in Group Versus Individual DPP Weight Loss Interventions – The SHINE Study. Diabetes.

28. Trimpey, J. (1996). *Rational Recovery: The New Cure for Substance Addiction*. Gallery Books. https://www.amazon.com/Rational-Recovery-Cure-Substance-Addiction/dp/0671528580.

29. Quinlan, N., Kolotkin, R., Fuemmeler, B., & Costanzo, P. (2009). Psychosocial outcomes in a weight loss camp for overweight youth. International journal of pediatric obesity : IJPO : an official journal of the International Association for the Study of Obesity.

30. Verified Market Research (2023, March 1). *Global Packaged Food Market Size By Material, By Product, By End-Use, By Geographic Scope And Forecast*. Retrieved June 25, 2023, from https://www.verifiedmarketresearch.com/product/packaged-food-market/#:

31. Wadden et al. (2005) found "The combination of medication and group lifestyle modification resulted in more weight loss than either medication or lifestyle modification alone." Wadden, T., Berkowitz, R., Womble, L., Sarwer, D., Phelan, S., Cato, R., Hesson, L., Osei, S., Kaplan, R., & Stunkard, A. (2005). Randomized trial of lifestyle modification and pharmacotherapy for obesity. The New England Journal of Medicine.

32. Willett, W.C., Wood, M., Childs, D., *Thinfluence*. Thin-flu-ence (noun) the powerful and surprising effect of friends, family, and environment have on weight. Rodale Press.

33. World Health Organization (2023, April 5). *Diabetes*. WHO.int. Retrieved May 31, 2023, from https://www.who.int/news-room/fact-sheets/detail/diabetes.

34. World Health Organization (2021, June 9). *Obesity and Overweight*. WHO. int. Retrieved May 31, 2023, from https://www.who.int/news-room/fact-sheets/detail/obesity-and-overweight.

35. World Health Organization (2021, June 11). *Cardiovascular Disease (CVD)*. WHO.int. Retrieved May 31, 2023, from https://www.who.int/news-room/fact-sheets/detail/cardiovascular-diseases-(cvds).

36. Wurtman, J.J. (2010). You Can Prevent PMS from Destroying Your Diet. [Blog post] Retrieved from https://www.psychologytoday.com/us/blog/the-antidepressant-diet/201008/you-can-prevent-pms-destroying-your-diet.

Printed in Great Britain
by Amazon

40568827R00106